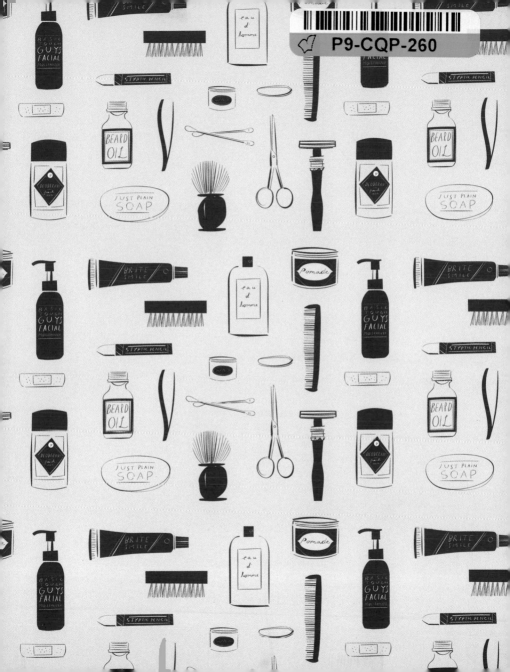

MAN
MADE

THE ART OF
MALE GROOMING

MAN
MADE

THE ART OF
MALE GROOMING

BY

DAN JONES

ILLUSTRATED BY LIBBY VANDERPLOEG

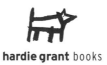

hardie grant books

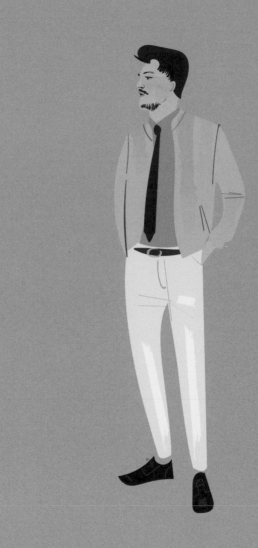

CONTENTS

INTRODUCTION

At 14 years old I was a real Ugly Betty. I had acne, train-track braces, a monobrow and wet-look 'fro. My yearbook photo shows a pained but smiling-through-it-all expression. By 16 my acne was even worse, and I'd graduated to styling my too-wavy hair into a hirsute helmet with just a hint of mullet. I found my first freak grey hairs when I was 19 – it happened almost overnight, like Rogue in *X-Men*. By then I had long locks, way past my shoulders, except it leapt out awkwardly in an angry cloud of frizz, as if it was trying to leave my head in search of a better life. I chopped it off and over the years experimented with some truly challenging looks: a mini-mohawk, spikes gunged with gel; I even shaved my head, only to expose a weird knobble at the back of my head like an extra nose.

But now, I think I look pretty good. By that I mean I worked out how to make the best of what I've got, and started to worry less about how I look.

As a former magazine editor, I've hit more than my fair share of grooming goals. I've tried and tested some tough treatments and upscale facials, had my face microwaved on Harley Street, and my love handles mishandled via a series of techy treatments that

Introduction

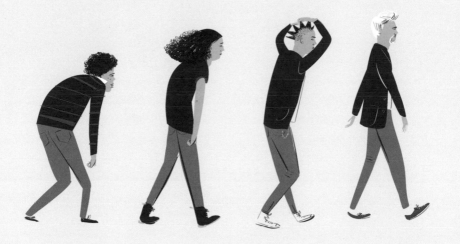

purported to melt them away. I've interviewed world experts on skincare, fitness and wellness; sat in the chair of the best barbers in the world; tried old-school wet shaves and intense sports massages. I've boot-camped and raw-cleansed, I've downward-dogged and powered through Pilates, waved glowsticks at a rave exercise class, even slut-dropped at a Beyoncé-themed dance fitness session. I've been inked by cult tattoo artists, pierced by piercers (it was the '90s – don't judge); I've front-rowed at fashion shows, worked with designers, stylists and photographers, and discovered what I look best in. I've studied which brands and items to invest in, and how best to look after my collection of clothes and shoes.

I'm not perfect. One of my cheeks is redder than the other (I look like I've been slapped if I have too much hot sauce on my *bánh mì*). I have fine lines, chicken pox scars; I'm sure that one of my eyes is a bit droopier than the other; and I'm forever in search of The Line – that impossible indentation running from sternum to belly button that appears when you've spent three hardcore months in the gym (and not evenings at home eating cake, watching box sets of *Game of Thrones*). And sometimes I wear my socks two days in a row.

All we can do is work with what we're given, try our very best and not be too self-focused about it all. And have a sense of humour about the things we can't change.

A great haircut, neatly trimmed beard, nails that are clean – clipped and clear of BBQ sauce, face exfoliated and moisturised, and award-winning personal hygiene are essential; then, a perfectly pressed shirt, well-fitting jacket and shiny shoes or fresh sneakers, and maybe some well-shaped glasses, if you need them. Add to that a good diet, a bit of exercise and a little stress control.

This book is for men and manly people of all ages – from teen upstarts to the ancient-and-awesome – and everyone in between. Even if you follow just a few of my recommendations, discoveries and hacks, you'll be firmly on your way to being just that little bit more epic. Man, made.

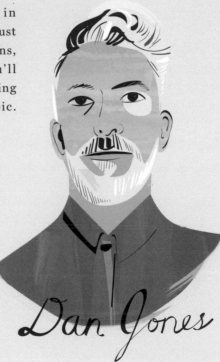

Dan Jones

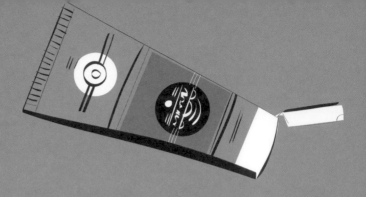

Chapter One
The Face

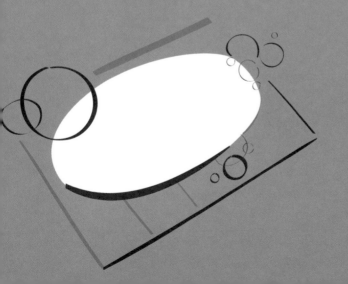

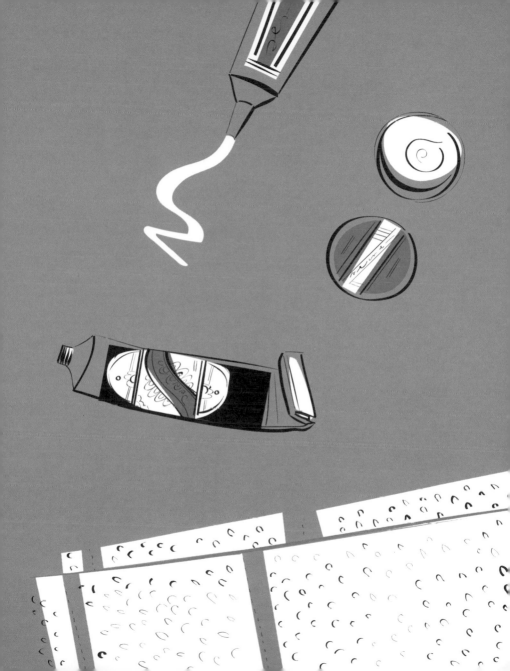

Man Made

Unless you go around wearing a gimp mask
zipped up over your head, your face is the first thing
people see. Yet, oddly, it's the last thing most men think
about. Many of us don't even use a basic moisturiser, or
bother with sunblock. We wash our face with
hand soap and shower gel.
Treat your face well and you'll preserve its firmness,
smoothness and all-round handsomeness, all the
way through to your later years. Treat it badly and –
before long – it will start to hang off your head like an
elephant's ball bag. The surprise here is that it's really
not hard to achieve a healthy tone, with minimal marks
and blemishes, and keep wrinkles and saggy bits at bay.
You just need to know your skin type, a few how-to tips,
and stick to a simple daily routine. That's the thing with
skin: you need to look after it. Like most things in life, it
works best when you keep it clean and protected.

KNOW YOUR SKIN TYPE

Pay attention, this is important. Knowing the type of skin you have and how it changes in different environments is key to how you treat your face, which products you choose and – ultimately – how you look.

Use the wrong product and it's like filling up your car with unleaded when it takes leaded. You should be using products based on what your face really needs. But how do you get personal with your skin type?

Examine your skin at the end of the day – that way a good few hours of wear and tear will show, oily sebum might have leaked onto your skin (particularly after lunch), and your chosen products will have all but worn off. Look at your T-zone (the T-shaped area of skin around your forehead and your nose) and see if it's too oily, too dry or somewhere happily in between.

NORMAL

You're looking for a soft, springy consistency, not too oily, and not too dry, but a slight rubbery feel. If this is you, you're a lucky, lucky man. You can usually use any product without fear of a freak breakout – but a bit of work (washing, exfoliating and more) is needed to keep things in balance.

OILY

You have anything from a light sheen of oil to a face like the bottom of a deep-fat fryer – and the accompanying blackheads and blemishes when it's out of control. Using oil-based products is a big mistake, especially for acne-prone skin. A simple fix is to look for lotions rather than creams. Try gels and clarifying products and avoid anything too rich. And make sure you exfoliate regularly as oily skin will attract dirt and grit more than other types.

DRY

Does your skin feel raspy and dry, even a little flaky like a sausage roll? You're dry, like

the best kind of wit. You are more likely to be prone to skin sensitivity, so natural, no-nasties products with rich moisturising properties are best. Use a cream rather than a lotion, and pay attention to the oil content – the higher the better.

COMBINATION

Oily forehead and nose, but curiously dry cheeks? You're a bit of both, my friend. Consider your skin bi-furious. It's a tricky one to buy for, as different areas respond in different ways to the same product. When in doubt, focus on oil-free products that are simple but nourishing.

Seasonal Tweaks

When it's very cold out, adjust your regime: miss out a few exfoliation sessions – your skin will be weather-beaten enough. Consider a gel if you're somewhere very humid, like that winter-sun trip to Thailand, or a stressful morning spent lost in a Marrakech hammam wearing only a towel (I speak from experience). Steamy environments, rich moisturisers

---

YOUR GROOMING ROUTINE

How to Wash Your Face

What is wrong with soap and water? Everything. Your average bar of soap is alkaline. While great at removing dirt, it tends to go even further, stripping your skin of moisture, leaving it tight and itchy. Washing your face should give you a clean slate – not dry out your skin, or leave it too oily. Pick a face wash that suits your skin type – use it little and often – and keep yourself looking tiptop.

THE LATHER

First, use a small amount of face wash to thoroughly clean your hands, then splash your face with lukewarm water. Next add a small amount of face wash to your fingertips and gently rub your face in a circular motion, working outwards from the centre, creating a lather. Try to give yourself at least 30 seconds – or more – to do this, paying special attention to your forehead and nose, and get in all the cracks and crevices. Don't forget your jawline and neck, your hairline and behind your ears. Most people don't spend enough time on the lather but 30+ seconds really does the trick. And it doesn't matter where you do it – the shower, the sink, on the bus – just so long as it becomes part of your routine.

A word of warning: don't be too rough. Your skin has to last the distance and treating it too roughly means that, over your lifetime, it could drift a little from its moorings and start to sag.

THE SPLASH OFF

After the lather, splash off the face wash with fresh lukewarm water. Make sure there's no residue, especially around your beard or moustache, the edges of your jaw or the temples, as a build-up of product can block pores and encourage breakouts.

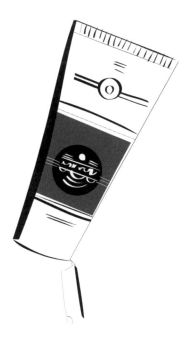

Although you don't need a washcloth, it's a good idea. Ever had a hot towel treatment at the barber's? Where you're wrapped up like the Invisible Man with a near-scorching damp towel that's fresh out of the autoclave? Then you'll know how utterly, mind-blowingly relaxing it feels. And when you're unwrapped, revealing dewy, flushed baby skin, it's like you're a newborn. Using a soft washcloth at home has something of a similar, invigorating, welcome-to-the-world effect.

THE DRY UP

A clean towel is pretty much essential. Too often I discover my 'clean' towel is actually the one I used to dry off my dog, Gary – although it's usually too late by the time I realise. Assuming this doesn't happen to you, just pat your face dry. Don't rub or scrub, which can damage your skin, just dab your face. And there

you are, fresh, clean and dry – and ready to absorb any other clever products you want to smear on.

PROBLEMS?

If you're using a mild, foaming face wash that still leaves you feeling tight every time, you're probably washing away moisture from your skin along with the city dirt and ketchup smears. Switch to a cream-based wash – it'll soften your skin and clean it at the same time. Combination skin? Use a cream wash in the morning and your foaming one at night to give your face a little balance. Ultimately, all skin types – even oily ones – need hydration and can benefit greatly from a little gentle cleansing.

Exfoliation

Once, maybe twice a week, you should exfoliate. The process of removing dead skin cells will leave

---

Icons of Grooming

MR NICK WOOSTER

The term 'Silver Fox' was almost definitely invented for Nickelson Wooster, whose perfectly styled silver hair and beard (which appears in various lengths and guises) and impeccable outfits cause the same brouhaha among street-style photographers outside fashion shows usually reserved for his female front-row counterparts. As fashion consultant, Instagram superstar, accessories designer and style savant, Wooster can score trillions of Likes wearing almost any outfit – from a bespoke three-piece suit to a crumpled pair of swim shorts and shirt. He just gets it. If you take any tip from Wooster, it's to be bold and brave – don't be afraid to experiment with your style, or underestimate the power of a good jacket.

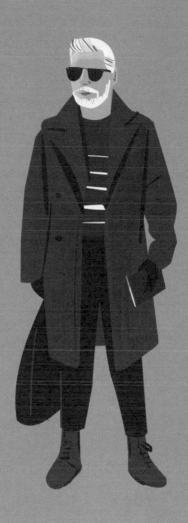

your skin looking and feeling fresher, cleaner and a whole lot smoother. Do it right and you'll be unclogging pores, shedding flaky skin, and uncovering hairs that might otherwise start to grow inwards, getting itchy and infected. Do it too enthusiastically and you are left with a face that is sensitive and sore – like that scene in *RoboCop* (the original, obviously) when the bank robber drives into a vat of toxic waste and his face melts off.

The good news is that it's easy to get right. You just need a facial cleanser that has a little grit in it (exfoliators contain anything from fruit seeds to ground-up pumice stone) – and then use it the same way you might apply your face wash. Squeeze some of the exfoliator onto the tips of your fingers and rub gently into the face using a circular motion, working out from the centre of your face, for 30+ seconds – with

a little lukewarm water to loosen things up.

Pay attention to the nose (and the little crevices either side) to make sure you're helping unclog all your pores. If you have more than a little light acne, you're best off using a specific (and very gentle) anti-bacterial exfoliator. Some products use a mild acid to help things along – salicylic, glycolic, alpha hydroxy and beta hydroxy acids often pop up on product labels, along with fruit enzymes and traditional exfoliating elements that range from sea salt to peach pits. Some are cream- or gel-based, some come as a powder, but they all pretty much achieve the same thing: great-looking skin.

I recommend something fairly mild – that scene from *RoboCop* haunts me – but the harshness of an exfoliating product is personal preference. The question is, how gritty do you like it?

HOW TO MOISTURISE

You've cleansed your face and patted it dry with a clean towel, so now – while your skin is in this moist, receptive state – you can apply your moisturiser. Apply small dabs to your cheekbones, forehead and chin; and don't forget your neck. Like using a face wash, gently smooth over your skin in a circular motion with your fingertips, moving out and up. Watch out for any residue caught at the edges of your face or lodged in your beard, and make sure all your moisturiser gets fully absorbed. Ideally, try to apply moisturiser twice a day: in the morning and before you go to sleep. Some of us find this a little challenging, so applying just once – after your morning shower – should also do the trick.

The Right Ingredients

Your moisturiser – matched to your skin type – should be rich in all the right ingredients: oils, botanical extracts, antioxidants, even UVA and UVB sunblock, with

How to Pick Your First Tattoo

No dolphins, yin-yangs, Chinese symbols you don't understand; no infinity symbols or clusters of stars sparkling across your abs; no flocks of birds or Celine Dion lyrics. Tattoo art has its trends: those wincingly bad barbed-wire or tribal tattoos you now see hanging flaccid off someone's arm? They were cool once. Fact. Your first tattoo is perhaps the gravest, most important decision of your life – or so it seems at the time. Months of research into images and artists and esoteric symbols until it's finally inked onto your skin – and then it's all about having another, anything, and how soon: it's easy to get hooked. Thing is, you are picking a new permanent feature of your body, so you need to feel comfortable with whatever you get: its shape, colour and angle, the longevity of its style, and what it represents (you'll need to defend it when necessary). Shop around, research the artist and studio, and pick a tattooist who has real experience in the type of image you're after. Finally, watch your spelling, punctuation and subordinate clauses.

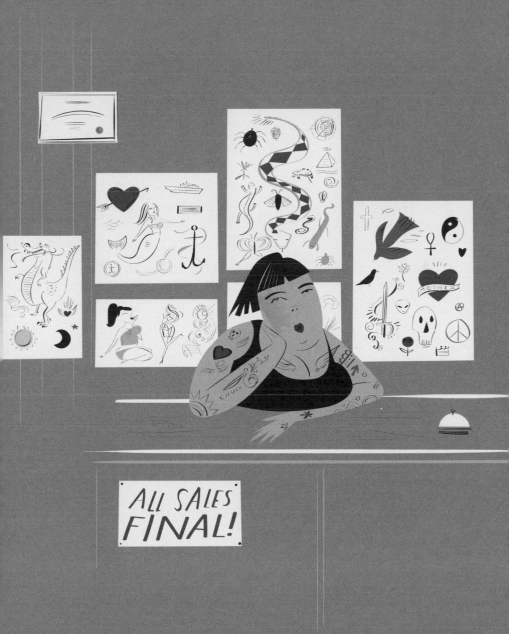

a few little power-boosters like caffeine or vitamins and minerals. Here's what to look out for:

OILS

Modern moisturisers contain a combination of oily extracts – anything from coconut, jojoba and almond to hemp, avocado, rosemary, argan, ylang-ylang and more. These are blended into clever cocktails that power up products with special qualities to even out your skin's own natural oiliness.

SHEA BUTTER

The fatty, oily substance extracted from the nut of the shea tree is known for its thick, rich texture and strong hydrating properties. It's a natural source of vitamin A, and its make-up is similar to the oils your own skin makes.

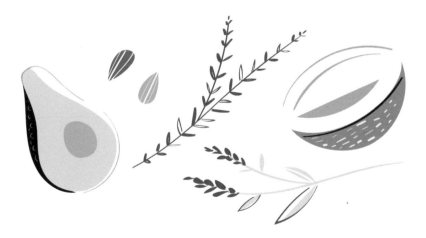

So, in theory, it should sink easily into the skin.

FRIENDLY ACIDS

Alpha hydroxy acids increase exfoliation and the shedding of skin cells – useful if you're looking for even-toned, smooth skin. Look for glycolic acid and lactic acid. Salicylic acid works similarly and can help keep your pores clear. Omegas are fatty acids that are brilliant at moisturising the skin.

GLYCERIN

An important fat that can be plant-derived or created synthetically. Glycerin is a humectant, which means it magically draws water from the air onto your skin and forms a protective layer to stop moisture getting out.

It's a tiny bit controversial; when used in a very dry environment, where there's not a whole lot of moisture in the air, it seems to pull moisture up out of the skin's deeper layers, drying it out. But when it's used with the right ingredients it's a powerful element in a moisturiser.

SILICONE

Another water-binding agent, silicone is sometimes used in moisturisers to offer protection from the elements. Products that contain too much silicone can leave your face looking a bit shiny, so use with a little caution.

ANTIOXIDANTS

No one wants to oxidise like last night's bowl of guacamole, but that's just what your skin's doing right now (albeit very slowly). Antioxidants – often extracted from botanical treatments – are clever little molecules that we still don't know that much about, apart from the fact that they seem to delay cell damage. Green tea is an excellent source of antioxidants, along with grape seed, coffee berries, vitamin C and phloretin (found in apples).

SUN PROTECTION

A few years ago I interviewed Dr Leslie Baumann, one of the world's most accomplished skin specialists. She's based in Miami, the tropical sunshine city of crazy humidity (where people shop in tiny fluoro bikini briefs and roller boots – and that's just the guys), which might explain her strong focus on sun protection. She was emphatic that it's one of the most important skincare essentials we should be using every single day – even in winter. And who are we to argue?

There are two types of skin-damaging rays that you need to know about: UVA (ultraviolet A) and UVB (ultraviolet B). UVA ages the skin, but in a way we can't see obviously at the time, whereas UVB burns – and it's

pretty obvious when it does. Most sunscreens are UVB-proof, but not all protect against UVA, so you should always check if it is mentioned on the packaging. If it's not on there, then it won't protect against ageing. If you have oily skin, skip your usual moisturiser. Otherwise, apply SPF first, wait for it to settle, then add moisturiser as a topcoat.

Following the Rules

Those 'how to use' directions on the back of the bottle? They actually mean something. If you're not following the rules, you're sabotaging your products. Use them correctly and store them appropriately. Placing your kit in a cupboard next to hot water pipes or a medicine cabinet over a light fitting will gently slow-cook it, decreasing its potency.

TROUBLESOME SKIN PROBLEMS: TEEN TO MATURE

ACNE

Its medical name, aptly, is acne vulgaris. It usually debuts proudly at puberty but can carry on, or even make a late appearance, all the way through adulthood too. Your skin contains sebaceous glands that pump out sebum, the oily substance that coats and protects the skin. But when your skin becomes unbalanced (due to irritation, infection, allergies or raging pubescent hormones) too much sebum is produced. Then the fun begins: hair follicles become blocked, and dead skin, dirt and debris clump together, providing the ideal hangout spot for bacteria. You get pain and swelling underneath the blockages that cause anything from the odd zit to a full-blown acne party on your face. Raised, sore lumps; whiteheads (small, hard bumps with a white centre); pustules packed with pus; even nodules (hard painful lumps under the skin) are all potential guests. The trickiest is inflammatory acne, which affects large swathes of your skin and can leave scarring. Treating acne is personal to the host – smart combinations of products and a special skincare routine can really help, and eating chocolate or a KFC bargain bucket has little effect.

CAN YOU SQUEEZE ZITS?

The official line is: no, don't squeeze them. But in reality, most dermatologists know it's just too tempting not to. Generally, if the centre is white or yellow, you can probably pop it. Consider it a surgical procedure: have scrupulously clean hands, clipped nails and a washed face. Use two cotton buds and press down around the zit. Don't push the cotton buds towards each other;

you could force the crud down further into your skin, making the situation much worse. Once you've teased out the pus, stop and stand back to admire your work. Most people make things worse when they pop, and doing it obsessively can lead to scarring, so enjoy those few moments of mastery.

REDNESS

Anyone can get rosacea, but it's usually those with light skin who suffer the most. If you blush easily, or get a flushed face when drinking alcohol or eating chilli, you might be prone to a little facial redness later in life. It is caused by tiny veins in the face becoming enlarged, giving you a flushed appearance. It usually pops up on the cheeks, forehead, nose and chin, and it can be intermittent at first, before it settles into a more permanent state, sometimes with pimples and bumps. There's a school of thought that suggests rosacea is genetic in nature, but there are treatments to reduce or eradicate it (ask your doctor) and there are some simple steps to help the appearance. You should avoid the sun, alcohol and spicy foods – all of which could dilate the blood vessels, making any redness look worse.

BLACKHEADS

What sort of person obsessively watches hundreds of YouTube videos of uncensored blackhead squeezing? Me. It's become a hobby of mine, my peccadillo, if you will. The anticipation of the big squeeze... and then the POP! Exciting times. What I've learnt is that they're incredibly tempting to squeeze. They're open to the air (unlike whiteheads) and – sometimes – tend to slip out without much effort. Also, they respond brilliantly to products that contain salicylic acid, which helps to exfoliate and unblock your pores. Salicylic can be harsh in high quantities, so be careful when using washes and creams that contain it. Avoid benzoyl and hydrogen peroxide – both are effective on proper pus-filled zits, but they're not so hot on blackheads. Exfoliate regularly, and try a pore strip (stick-on strips that tug tens of blackheads out at a time in a rather dramatic and satisfying way).

WRINKLES

Just accept them. Perhaps that's a little controversial, given the many gazillions of dollars spent on researching, producing and marketing anti-ageing products, but, honestly, they're just a part of growing older. Plus, in a patriarchal society, where women are told they must look young forever, men get to look 'distinguished'. There are very

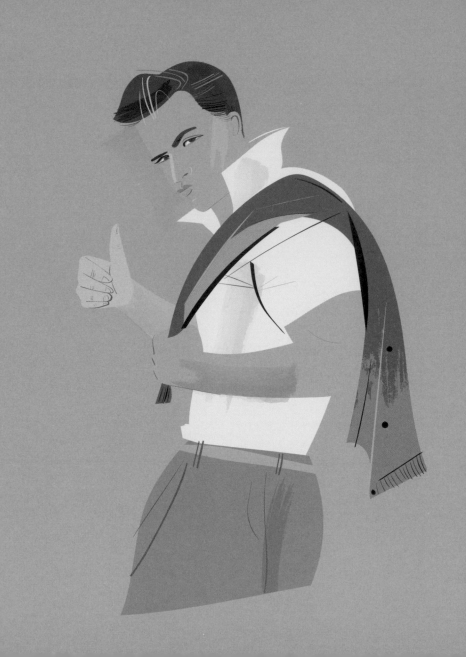

How Not to Look Like a Dick in a Photo

Think about the best thing that has ever happened to you. Think about when you were happiest. Perhaps it involved pizza? Now, let that memory shoot out of your eyes like laser beams; let it stretch a smile across your face and make you stand up straight, shoulders back, belly tucked in.

There are many ways not to look like a dick in a photo, but feeling nothing less than amazing usually does the trick. Wear what you feel great in. Maybe stand at a slight angle to the camera, check your lighting (make sure it's not at the side, or shining up creepily from below; natural is best) and – this is the clincher – try not to pose. If you really must, try out a few looks on your own, pick the best and call on your trademark photo face whenever it is required. No hip-pops, please. And you know where you can put your selfie stick.

few topical, over-the-counter treatments to combat fine lines and wrinkles, and none that effectively – and exceptionally – reverse ageing. So, it's more a case of prevention, and then acceptance when they finally arrive. If you're able to, look to your parents and grandparents to see what's coming down the track and pre-empt problems as your skin matures. With sun damage sometimes taking years – decades, even – to visibly affect the skin, it's a good idea to do a little bit of reconnaissance.

TREATMENTS & TECH

Non-Invasive

No needles or knives allowed – just expert facials, electrifying tonal treatments (which purport to tone up muscles and improve skin quality), enzyme packs and collagen masks. The non-invasive skin-treatment industry is both complicated and expensive, but some therapies do actually work. I'd try out something non-invasive over anything that cuts into your skin. And so should you.

MICRODERMABRASION

It's the super-powered version of exfoliation, with a lightly abrasive planing tool or crystal-packed exfoliant and a machine that gently sucks away debris, followed by some cooling ointment to soothe irritated skin. Think of it as a bit like removing plaque from your teeth at the dentist, but without the minty fresh finish and rude receptionist.

CHEMICAL PEELS

A chemical solution is painted onto your face, making the top layer blister and shed off like a snake. It sounds horrific, doesn't it? And you'll look pretty scary while it's happening. Superficial peels are left on for a few minutes and your skin might feel a bit tight afterwards – and the downtime isn't as long.

Middle-strength peels remove the upper and middle layers of skin; if you have light skin it might turn red or brown in the days after the peel, and it can take up to six weeks for your skin to turn back to normal. Deep peels get right down to the bottom of the epidermis and you might need an anaesthetic to take the edge off. Ultimately, you're damaging your skin, killing off the top layer and therefore encouraging new growth underneath. It had better be worth it.

Botox & Fillers

The muscle-paralysing toxin botulinum has been part of grooming and beauty culture for years. Botox relaxes facial muscles and makes wrinkles less obvious; it's injected in freehand by a doctor and effects start to become evident after a few days, or as long as two weeks, staying that way for at least three-to-four months. Want to fix one part of your face? Smoothing out your forehead wrinkles, say, might highlight other areas of your face that could also do with a little work. You might end up having more Botox than you bargained for, giving you that frozen, lightly greased look. Dermal fillers are injections used to fill out wrinkles and crevices in the skin, pumping it up like a baker's piping bag. They're made from a variety of materials and the effects can be either temporary or permanent, depending on the type of filler.

Tried & Tested: Red Alert

I once had my face microwaved on Harley Street in London.

A thread vein treatment that purported to zap away fine veins and redness and not leave it looking like an angry slapped arse. My whole family tends to have a bit of a ruddy complexion, and a red blotchiness had started to spread across one of my cheeks and the bridge of my nose. Drinking a Dirty Martini would turn it from a faded blush to clown's-nose crimson.

The procedure was expensive, a little bit painful and carried out by a consultant who wore huge magnifying video-camera glasses. But ten minutes later I was out on the street and back to work. Weeks later the redness (which had increased initially) had settled down to a flamingo pink, and then faded to nothing. It balanced out the tone of my skin and the veins that had once been snaking across my face had all disappeared. Result.

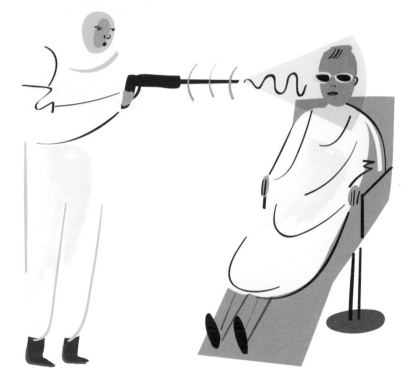

Icons of Grooming

MR PHARRELL WILLIAMS

When Naomi Campbell gives you grooming tips, you listen. Legend has it that the supermodel pulled him aside and told him to ditch cheap products and go to a dermatologist. Pharrell maintains that well-chosen inexpensive lotions and potions can be used with a bit of due diligence, but, at the end of the day, you just have to 'look after your face'. And that's just what he's done. As he enters his early 40s, the artist, designer and fragrance creator champions the idea of dressing how you feel – and not to force it. That, and SpongeBob socks.

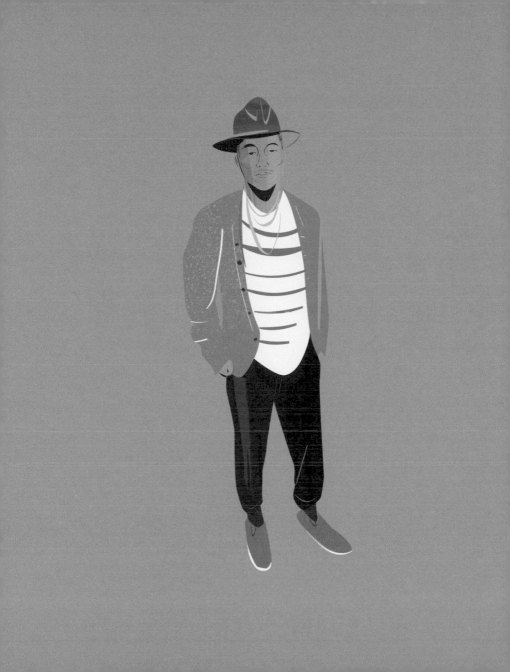

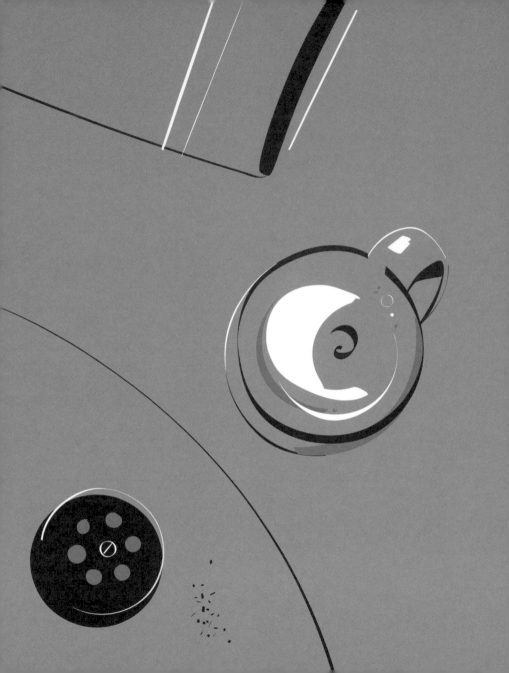

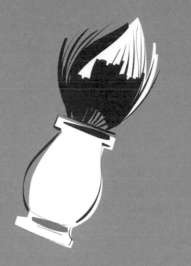

Chapter Two

The Shave

Clean and pristine through to full pelt, the sliding scale of facial hair allows for all manner of variations: closely shaven to jaunty moustache to unkempt, wild-man beard – and everything in between. Shave properly and your skin won't let you down. Grow moustaches and beards with a few inside tips, and more than a little bravery.

HOW TO SHAVE

Legend has it that your dad teaches you to shave. But what if Dad wasn't around? Maybe he was working on an oil rig, or travelling the land selling ladies' undies from a suitcase, and you were left to work out your own shaving routine? Even if you did learn a thing or two from your father, it's a good idea to reset and re-learn exactly how it's done. Thankfully, it's surprisingly simple.

THE WASH

Wash your face – using your usual face wash – and make sure your beard is damp and soft. (For this reason, shaving after you shower is optimal.)

THE LATHER

Add shave foam, cream, gel or oil, and massage in with your fingertips, making sure every hair is covered. If you have sensitive skin – or a very thick beard – let the product sink in for a moment; you want your beard to be as soft and supple as possible. Here's where you might like to use the retro combo of a brush, shaving soap and mug – floating in hot water in a full sink to keep the lather nice and warm. (Though this is not essential.)

THE SHAVE

Using a clean multi-blade razor, gently shave with the grain of the hair. Use light pressure, rinsing the blade with warm running water after each stroke. Pull your skin taut to decrease drag, and work your way around the face and neck. Be aware of the razor angle – don't make it too steep. The blade should cut through the hair easily; there's a tendency to increase the angle as the razor loses its sharpness, but it's far better just to replace the blade. Rinse well with cold water to help seal your pores, and pat dry.

Foams, Gels, Creams & Oils

Foams, creams and gels offer a hydrating richness to your skin and beard, and – as they're transparent – oils are perfect if you have any lumps and bumps on your skin that you want to avoid shaving. I almost always recommend using a product made for sensitive skin, even if yours is particularly tough. Shaving damages your skin. Although skin can recover quickly, shaving is an invasive practice that can cause real irritation. Oils aren't just recommended for those who want to see what they're shaving, and you don't have to use them on their own – they'll power up a shaving foam if applied underneath.

Razors

Spend a little money here – a high-quality, sturdy razor makes all the difference between nicks, cuts, your face looking like a warzone, and a smooth, even shave. So, what's best? Disposables? Multi-blade razors? Safety razors? Straight razors?

Let's start with what's worst. Single-blade disposables can rip your face to shreds. Don't even think about it.

Multi-blade razors are usually excellent. I'm loath to recommend a single brand, especially one that's not particularly cheap, but Gillette makes a rather good multi-blade razor. Drawbacks are that hair can get clogged between the blades, and they're pricey, but they're exceptional and hard to misuse.

Safety razors are those metal, vintage-looking razors that hold a single blade in a safety compartment – and which you can also change manually. They are a little fiddly at times, but as long as the blade is of sufficient quality, a safety razor is a dream to use. Plus, buy a sturdy brand – like a Merkur or an Edwin Jagger – and it will probably last you a lifetime.

Straight razors are the Sweeney Todd of the family. There's an art to it, a special way to hold it, and a unique angle (30 degrees) to achieve. The results are much the same as other razors – it's more the ancient ritual of it all that's the draw here. For me, it's a bit too retro for retro's sake and has no real edge on the competition, plus the chance of nicks and cuts is high. Although the extras – the shaving brush, for example – are worth remembering. Your call on whether you want to try a straight razor, if only for the experience.

Homemade Hot Towel

To ready your skin and soften your beard for shaving, take a clean flannel or small towel, add a few drops of an essential oil (lavender is thought to have anti-inflammatory properties) or menthol rub, fold over and douse with hot water from the tap; let it steep in boiled water straight from the kettle, or microwave it damp in a dish. Wait until it has cooled to a safe temperature, and then wrap it – steaming – around your face, barbershop style. It's probably one of the most relaxing sensations on the planet.

Wet v Dry

Dry shaving is a grooming crime. At least, that's what the razor manufacturers would have you believe. Certainly, wet shaving has a far greater success rate if you are aiming for a completely clean, very close shave. But a dry electric shaver can be pretty useful when on the run. Choose between foil and rotary mechanisms, and don't let your beard grow too long before using them (the hairs will get yanked out, painfully). Expect a great, close shave on the protruding parts of your face, but on your cheeks, and especially your neck, expect to find patches of hair the blades never touch.

Tried & Tested: Barbershop Shave

You must try this, at least once. The hot towel, the scrub-up, the lather, the artist's attention to detail as the straight or multi-blade razor glides over your face; even the glass of bourbon. It's a world-class feeling and you almost always look great – and I defy you not to fall asleep. Combine it with a trim for extra sharpness.

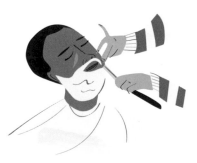

HOW TO WEAR A MOUSTACHE

Want to grow a meaty moustache, a porn-star handlebar, or a little trimmed tickler? I'm a big fan of the stealth method: the trick is to create the beginnings of a beard. A few days of stubble look far less out of place than a fluffy top lip that's weeks away from proper moustache realness. Shave clean – or trim – around it and start growing out your almost-moustache for another week or two before you begin to shape and style it.

I recommend trimming – very, very carefully – over the top lip; it shouldn't be hanging down, irritating your mouth, making it hard to eat BBQ ribs, or make you act like a street freak (absent-mindedly and obsessively licking your lips to satisfy the hairy tickle of a stray hair – I speak from experience). Comb it through with

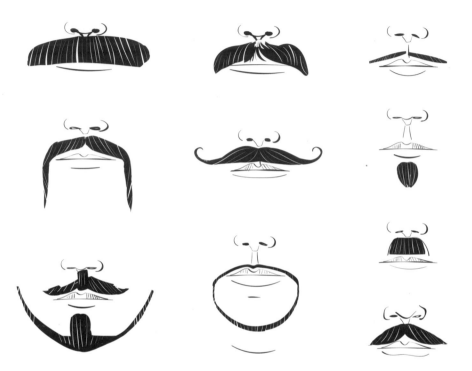

a fine-tooth comb and cut off any unruly hairs that spring up. If it's your first-ever moustache, get a barber to perform your first trim-and-shape session. The shaping and wearing of a moustache is art in reverse: it's more about the hair you remove than you leave. Think of your moustache (and beard) like the hair on your head. Wash it with

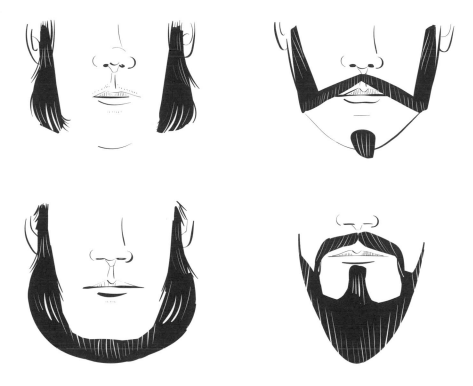

shampoo and condition it regularly; apply a little beard oil for softness (or coconut oil – a great grooming hack) and even a little moustache wax to retain shape and gloss.

THE HANDLEBAR CLUB

Founded in 1947, the world's premier moustache members' organisation, the Handlebar Club, is a monthly meet-up for the UK's moustachioed elite. Loiter around the bar at the Windsor Castle pub, London W1, every first Friday of the month and you'll see prime handlebars in their traditional habitat. The Handlebar Club is a friendly social network of moustache owners who gather to drink fine ales and talk some serious 'tache. No beards allowed.

HOW TO GROW A BEARD

The beard is a purely male domain. Not a wispy pre-teen type, but a nice thick hairy wedge. Growing your first is a little nerve-wracking. You anticipate a luxurious, lustrous bush, but what if all you can muster is a patchy, feeble smattering? No need to worry; it's not, perhaps, the beard itself that is the true badge of manhood but the strength of spirit required to grow one to fruition. It's a true rite of passage, ignoring taunts and sniggers, the screams of young relatives, and countless hair-based pitfalls such as discovering a whole new way to eat soup. It's worth it, though. Just look at history's bearded greats, like Marx, Ginsberg, Hagrid and Gandalf – their combined successes were woven into the very fabric of their impressive beards.

Are you a beard virgin? Don't tell anyone your ambitions. Just stop shaving and let it grow out for a good few weeks (most groomers recommend a full month at least) before you start to trim it into shape. Like a moustache, keep it clean as you would your hair (via a mild shampoo and conditioner) and apply a little beard oil to condition, or coconut oil. The first week is easy, the second, a little itchy as the hairs become long enough to turn around and irritate the skin. At the third week and beyond your new beard may have a slightly shaggy look – trimming the upper cheeks, top lip and neckline will improve its shape.

DON'T OVER-SCULPT

This is not 1998. Go against your instincts and let your beard grow down your neck a little. You'll want to trim it following the curve of your jawline, but it's almost impossible to do correctly without some help. Look head-on in the mirror and clipper or shave a straight horizontal line level with the point of your chin. It'll look a bit square at the edges, but it'll give your beard something to grow into. As with the moustache, if you are growing a beard for the first time, I'd recommend getting a barber to oversee that first trimming session. Then all you have to do is keep it in check. And pick cereal out of it when the time comes.

BRISTLY BEARD

At times, my beard feels like a scrubbing brush – usually after I've been swimming or out in the

How to Care for Your Beard

Think of it as a small pet – feed it, groom it and take it to the vet's (barber's) once in a while to keep it tiptop. Starting from scratch? Give it time to grow before your first grooming session (at least a week for the super-hirsute, and as much as six weeks for the less-hairy), and keep the skin in and around the beard clean and exfoliated – especially during the first couple of weeks to prevent ingrown hairs. There'll be a few itchy days when once-shaved hairs will curl back and tickle the skin with their spiky ends, but battle on. Then groom away with an adjustable beard trimmer – tidying up the edges with a razor – and use a trimming attachment or small scissors to clip away the hairs that dangle over your top lip. Wash it with a mild shampoo, use a little conditioner, and watch out for soap build-up. Oh, and continue to moisturise underneath your beard. Beard oil is a luxury – add a few drops before combing through – and the occasional trim at the barber's is essential.

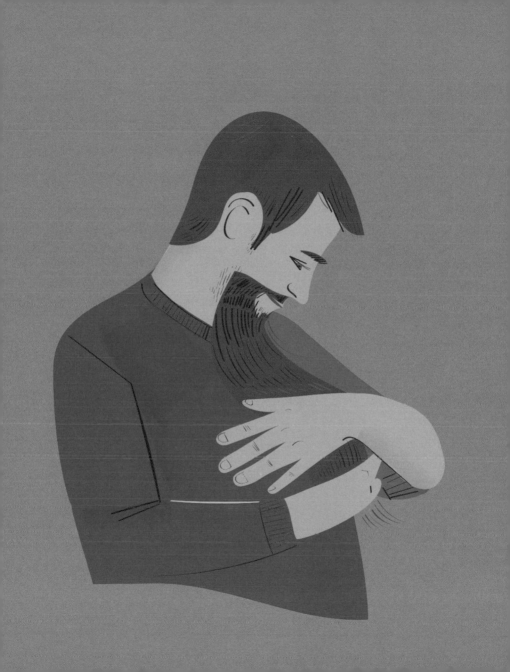

elements. It's at times like these that those seemingly superfluous grooming products come into their own.

Beard moisturiser is an actual product, and a rather clever buy. There are light products for super-short, three-day-old beards and thick, rich moisturisers for thick, rich beards. Oils are a worthy investment – scented with all sorts of manly fragrances; as is old-school brilliantine (such as that made by excellent grooming purveyors Taylor of Old Bond Street), a scented light oil that moisturises and refreshes with a little bit of shine. A beard balm – thicker than an oil – will build up softness: the perfect preventative of pash rash. But my personal recommendation is coconut oil: it's super-light, only very lightly fragranced and you can even fry bacon with it. Impressive stuff.

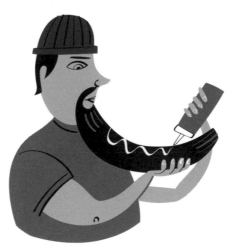

■

TROUBLESOME SHAVE PROBLEMS: TEEN TO MATURE

Ingrown Hairs

Ingrown hairs have curled around and – quite rudely – grown back into the skin. (It's the fine point shaving gives a single hair that renders it pointy enough to poke back into the skin.) They almost always bring a little bacteria with them and get infected; they're itchy and embarrassing and tend to occur if you have particularly curly or coarse hair. They're a little like zits in that they should usually be left alone to do their own thing. But dermatologists know that most people pick and squeeze their spots and blemishes, and an ingrown hair isn't any different. If you really, really must, clean up first, use sterilised tweezers or even a needle and some antiseptic ointment, and gently coax the hair out. Mild cases can clear up on their own, and shaving less closely – perhaps using a single-blade safety razor – can help. Ultimately, growing out your beard a little will give your skin time to calm down and heal.

Shaving Rash

To prevent the angry, sore and itchy skin discolouration you can get after shaving, exfoliate regularly, shave with a super-clean and sharp razor, and use gentle strokes, with a good splash of cold water at the end. A shaving brush can help when readying your beard for shaving – the bristles help each hair stand up straight, making them easier to cut with less drag. If your rash keeps reoccurring, consider changing your shaving routine – is your beard moist and supple enough? Do you need oil AND

gel or foam? And is your razor as sharp and clean as it can be?

Nicks & Cuts

It's actually quite difficult to cut yourself with a safety or multi-blade razor, but nicks happen. Washing and shaving brings blood to the surface of the skin, so any little shaving cut can bleed in seconds. Don't fancy stemming the flow with a tiny square of toilet paper? (Which is rather a good solution, if not a bit old school – so long as you remember to remove it before you head out for the day.) Add a styptic pencil to your grooming kit. It's an astringent in the shape of a lipstick. Wet the end and hold it against the nick for a few seconds to help constrict the tissues around the cut and stop the flow of blood. It stings, but it's worth it. Alum blocks – like a large salt lick – are soap-sized blocks of potassium alum, another astringent that you can wet and pass gently over your face. All out of toilet paper, styptic pencils and alum blocks? Cold water should do the trick.

NEVER SHAVE AGAIN

Sensitive skin, ingrown hairs and acne in my teens saw me give up wet shaving soon after I began. I invested in a set of clippers – the posh kind – and clipped my beard to a stubbly length: not quite a beard, and not clean shaven, but somewhere in between. My zits and shaving rash cleared up in days. I'd clipper two to three times a week – but it wouldn't matter if I missed a slot – and I'd wet shave now and then, usually for a special occasion. Now I waver between clippering, wet shaving (correctly, nowadays) and – as I write this – growing a grey beard, like Santa. If your skin problems are too pronounced and you're not warming to the idea of a beard, then clippering is the answer.

Icons of Grooming

MR PHILIP CRANGI

Many have tried but few have achieved Philip Crangi's facial hair perfection. The jewellery designer's grizzly look combines thickness and glossiness with perfectly performed grooming. And he mops it up after beer-drinking and sandwich-eating with one of his many vintage bandanas (how cool is that?). Also famous for his tattoos (he has 'Je ne regrette rien' across his chest), and he smells good too – if this illustration were scratch and sniff, it would smell of patchouli. What's not to love?

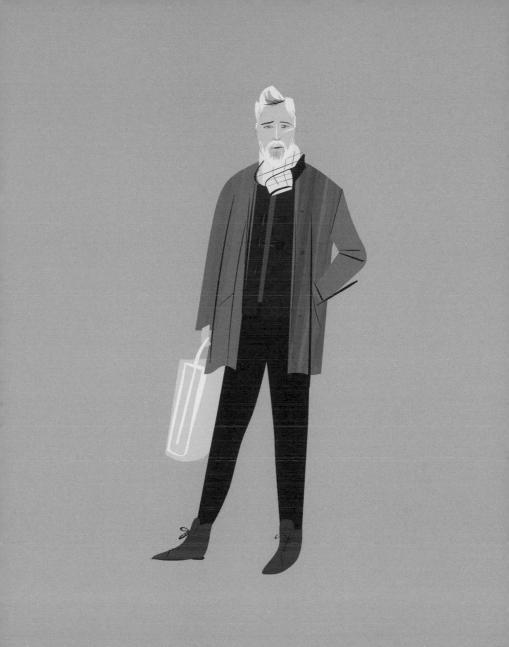

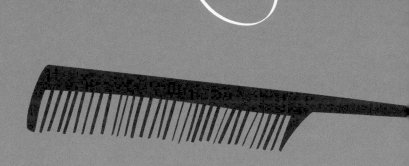

Chapter Three
The Hair

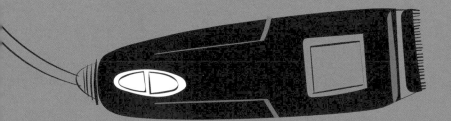

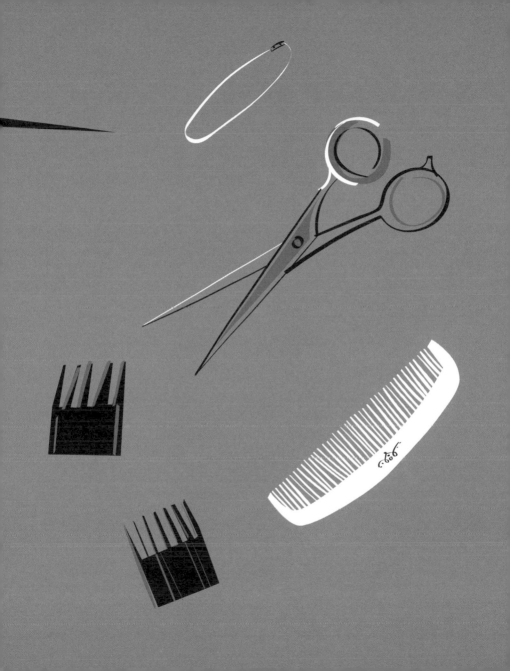

Are you sitting down? I have some bad news. Your hair is dead. DEAD. Each follicle is 100 per cent alive and kicking. But the strand itself? Stone-cold dead. That's why the job of keeping it in tiptop condition is so important. Because it's not going to wash, condition and style itself – it only looks as good as the effort you put into it. Spring to winter, as the elements strip important nutrients from your hair, it's up to you to fix it. Think of yourself as a hair mortician, if you will. Good news, then, that it's pretty easy to look after: identify your hair type and how it behaves in certain conditions, what styles suit it best, and pick the right hair goop to help get your mane in check.

KNOW YOUR HAIR TYPE

Density, coarseness and – um – shape of shaft are all factors in determining your hair type. It is easy to tell the difference between straight and curly, but what about the characteristics and behaviours particular to your crowning glory?

STRAIGHT

Is your hair stick-straight? Or does it have a slight wave adding a little volume when you grow it long? Either way, you have classic straight hair. Predictable, easy to cut and style, although a little flat and prone to oilines, it can be anything from super-fine to thick and coarse. Almost all cuts suit straight hair, but it really lacks volume. Those gravity-defying pompadours will need some architectural coaxing, industrial blow-drying and finger-crossing to stay upright.

WAVY

Anything from subtly wavy hair to a barnet teeming with S-shaped waves, or even some spiral curling when long, wavy hair ranges from super-fine to thick and coarse – although fine-to-medium coarseness and subtle waviness is pretty much perfect – you can have any of the cuts super-straight hair suits, but you'll have the body to achieve more exciting styles. Side parts, short and messy, even long, surfer beach bum all suit wavy hair.

CURLY

From big spiral curls to loose, natural waves and ringlets, right up to tight corkscrew curls, curly hair ranges from super-fine to thick and coarse. Super-tight curls look great at a short length (about 4 cm/2 in) and are best styled using your fingers rather than a brush or comb. A leave-in conditioner and styling creams – rather than gels or waxes – really bring out the best in your hair. Use a wide-tooth comb or just your fingers to comb through and style.

SUPER-THICK

Your hair is straight, wavy or curly, but its standout feature is that it is really thick – like a stallion's mane. Think of yourself as the centaur of the hair world. Thinning shears – those toothed barbershop scissors – can chop out the weight but often leave hair frizzy and, if used too close to the scalp, can create short hairs that stick up. Keep it well conditioned.

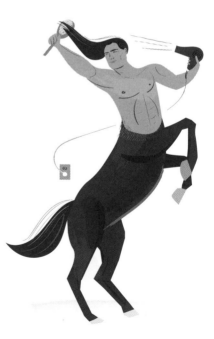

HOW TO WASH YOUR HAIR

Pick the right shampoo for your hair type, rinse your hair with warm water (not too hot), apply a large coin-sized dollop of shampoo and massage into your head using your fingertips. Give it a minute or two, concentrating on stimulating and exfoliating your scalp. Some say that this brings blood to the surface of the skin, nourishing your hair follicles which could slow down hair loss – but it's great for your scalp either way. Rinse, squeeze out the water, and then add your conditioner. If you're bearded (good for you), and your shampoo is mild, you can treat your bristles at the same time. Rinse and gently towel-dry – rubbing too vigorously in a circular motion will grind and damage your hair, and make it oily. Be gentle with your mane.

Tried & Tested: Co-Washing

If you have thick, wavy hair or super-curly coils, then washing your locks too often can create supersonic frizz and dryness.

You'll need more moisture than most, so experiment with ditching your shampoo for a few days and just condition and rinse. Look for co-wash cleansers and use a touch of hair powder to dry things up, if you need it. I tried it when my hair was particularly long and it worked a treat. I used shampoo every three-to-four days.

GOOP, AND HOW TO USE IT

Waxes, pomades, clays, gels and creams... Which one do you pick? Well, most of these have distinct differences, and some of them are modern inventions muscling in on old territory. Here's what you need to know about buying and using goop.

POMADE

In the 1800s, the main ingredient in pomade was bear fat or lard. But don't let that put you off. Usually petroleum-based, it is perfect for a slick, well-groomed retro cut; pomade is the high-shine product with real staying power.

The Hair

With different levels of intensity, strong versions work like a thick grease that, when added to wet or dry hair, can deliver all-day results – even in rainy conditions. Comb it through and style with a fine- or wide-tooth comb and the tracks will still be visible at the end of the day. The oily, almost wet look darkens hair, and it's tricky to wash out – it might even take a few goes. Pomade devotees merely rinse daily and reapply before a weekly shampoo. Also, it will trash your pillows. Lighter, water-based versions are easier to wash out and much more pliable. Oh, and watch out for goop slime – when your product starts to melt down onto your forehead throughout the day in hot climates. Not a great look.

WAX

Traditionally, wax was the matte-look alternative to pomade, but contemporary products can be just as glossy. Think of it as the middle point between pomade and gel: it's far more pliable, easier to apply and has a lighter hold on your hair. Pomade fights to force your hair into a style, wax works with your natural shape to improve it. It's great for oily hair as it washes out easily and rarely leaves a residue, and sometimes dries out within a few hours allowing you to restyle later in the day. It's not 100 per cent waterproof so might slip and slide off in the rain.

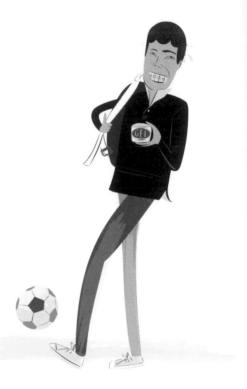

GEL

My PhD in hairology (i.e. the internet) tells me there is evidence that a hair gel-like substance was used in ancient Egypt, and in Iron Age times tree resin was also used to set some rocking styles. Whatever its manly history, it is usually the first hair product a teenager ever buys – I know that I thought supermarket own-brand wet-look hair gel looked awesome with train-track braces and acne. Contemporary gels are a little more refined, but in general the product sets your hair rock solid – there's little to no movement after you've styled it. The look is similar to using high-shine pomade, but gel washes or brushes out extremely easily. Best applied to damp hair.

CLAY & PUTTY

Hair clay and putty are marketed as premium hair products but work in much the same way as wax. They're easy to work with and produce texture and hold with a distinct matte finish. Apply to slightly damp hair and use your fingertips to style.

HAIR POWDER

When it is marketed to women, hair powder is called dry shampoo and it's usually – rather cleverly – in an aerosol can. For men, it's made to look like talc for the hair and scalp, soaking up oil and leaving no powdery trace. There are different colours to experiment with but a good honest everyman version in classic off-white should work just fine, even on super-dark hair.

HAIR CREAM

For the wavy-haired: this should be your key product. With its slight shine and simple light hold, it makes your hair look healthy and natural. In fact, it can look as if you're not wearing any product at all – which can be rather a good thing. Easy to apply, it should condition your hair throughout the day. Apply to damp hair, with optional Double Tap: apply a little more cream when your hair has dried to lock down your style. It's my product of choice.

Icons of Grooming

MR JUSTIN O'SHEA

Justin O'Shea has been street-style snapped more times than most, and with good reason – the Australian fashion buyer's slick-back hair, clipped beard, sunglasses, and rough-edged tatts (usually exposed via short, rolled-up sleeves) contrast perfectly with his clean, classic and upscale outfits. He seems to ignore flash-in-the-pan trends and sticks to iconic pieces: three-piece suits, shirts, leather shoes, and almost always a waistcoat. For O'Shea, it's all about looking good, but not showing off.

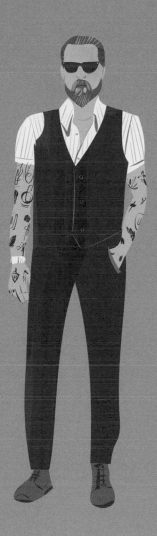

GOOP TIP: THE DOUBLE TAP

Grooming tradition decrees that product should almost always be applied to dry hair. Ignore this. Add a little styling cream to damp hair – let it dry naturally – and then finish off with a little more product. You'll get a deeper, stronger hold from hair that has dried with product combed through it, and increased shine and sharpness from adding a little more at the end. It's the Double Tap.

THE HAIR GALLERY

#1: THE FADE

If you ask for a Fade – the 1950s- influenced-yet-somehow-totally-modern cut – be prepared for your barber to whip out a switchblade and look you dead in the eye before he sets to work transforming you into a Belgian army cadet. He'll clipper off your hair super-short, about an inch above the ear, working around the entire head with mini-trimmers, or even a cut-throat razor to achieve a sharp, fresh look. It's a cut that takes a huge amount of skill; visit a barber who cuts Fades all day long. The process is repeated on the next section directly above the last-clipped area, changing the clipper setting up a notch, and so on. Finally, it's blended to achieve a subtle Fade, and hair on top is cut last. Variations are the Low Fade with long hair, or the super-tough-looking High and Tight, with a short crop on top that is less army cadet, more regional nightclub bouncer. The world's finest Fade cutter is arguably French barber, Mr Ducktail, who is based in London but cuts

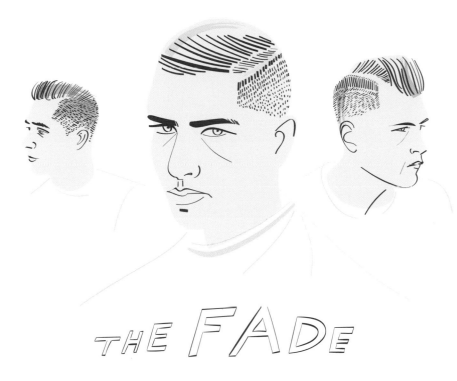

THE FADE

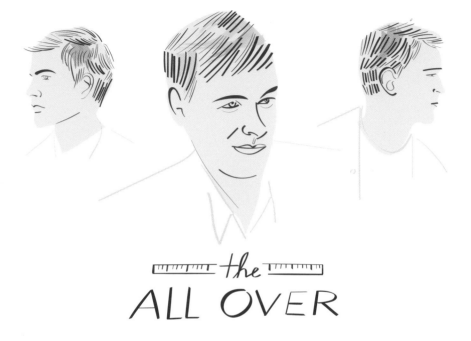

the
ALL OVER

all over the world. He only barbers hair strictly according to 1950s bad-boy styles (using his own-brand cola-scented hair grease), sometimes using a switchblade – earning him the nickname the Motherkutter. He has a fiercely loyal fanbase of hardcore rockabilly guys, and there is often a queue of tough-nuts outside, whichever store he is cutting in, even before it opens up.

#2: THE ALL OVER

The anti-style. The All Over is just what it claims to be: a one-length cut, that is usually achieved with clippers and is pretty much the same length all over. Zero skill is involved (you could even do it at home) and it looks best very closely cropped to the head with a little product for a nice, healthy shine. This is the cut my dad insists on getting – along with most men of a certain age – because it's utilitarian, easy and (more than a little) traditionally manly looking; but it has little-to-no style. Asking your barber to do this is a crime – would you ask a celebrated chef to ignore years of training and creative skill and just slam a tray of frozen chicken nuggets into the oven? In fact, that's a good way of thinking of the All Over – it's the chicken nugget of haircuts. But that's not to say you shouldn't wear it: there's a certain strength in having an All Over; it's almost a political statement, an eschewing of style in favour of something much more manageable and predictable. Think of the freedom in not worrying about how you look in the wind, rain, or after you've crawled out of bed! So, the All Over is a little bit chicken nugget, a little bit utilitarian, and a little bit 'Dad' in between.

#3: THE MAN BUN

The Man Bun, or Mun – the loose, not-quite-a-topknot bun of hair that's worn high at the back of the head – sharply divides opinion everywhere across the world, from backwater barbershops to high-end haircutters.

Like most male hair trends, it is – in part – celebrity-driven and, with a digital fanbase and whole Tumblrs and obsessive blogs devoted to it, for every bun-lover, there's a hater. In the style press, its detractors (usually the gruff, bald-headed variety) express concerns over its manliness, including the use of bands or clips to keep it in place, as if a Man Bun

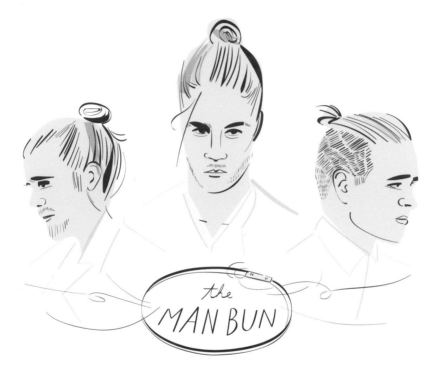

the
MAN BUN

automatically requires a crushed velvet scrunchie.

For all this feverish outrage, the Man Bun's main crime seems to be something so controversial it is completely at odds with society's perception of how men should wear their hair: buns are FUN. They are the diametric opposite of a short back and sides, or super-sharp Fades, but instead perch on your head like a wonky, hairy bird's nest. There's something wonderfully unkempt about them – a significant sense of rebellion, that at any moment you could ping off your elasticated band and let your hair spring out like Slash from Guns N' Roses.

To some, the Man Bun is the best men's hair trend ever to grace the head, and to others it's a slippery slope that ends with braided beards, crimped bangs, and frosted bubble perms. Whatever you think of the Man Bun, it's probably not something to get hot and cross over.

TROUBLESOME HAIR PROBLEMS

Losing It

Are you totally losing it? Is your hairline making a slow retreat, steadily increasing the distance between it and your eyebrows? Maybe there is the beginning of a tiny, shiny little bald patch at the back that no one thought to warn you about? Firstly, it's not necessarily a sign of ageing: lots of men in their 20s and 30s – even their teens – start to go bald. It's not the result of too much cheap hair gel, stress and sunburn, or not eating the crusts of your bread. Secondly, it's not always a side effect of having more than your fair share of testosterone (although some studies seem to suggest it is). You're merely genetically predisposed to being a baldy and it happens to about 50 per cent of us, and there's not a whole lot you can do about it. So you may as well bid it farewell in style... You don't have to wear a toupé or shave it all off – it's not the law (whereas a comb-over is indeed an international crime), and it could take 15 to 20 years to happen. Switching to a super-short cut – or maybe experimenting with a Fade – can make all the difference, as the top will seem all the thicker. Using a little product can tame fluffy, fine hair. And keeping your scalp clean, free of build-up and exfoliated can help keep your remaining hair follicles in tiptop condition. Ultimately, you might want to think about your approach to going bald; it's a natural process. And you never know – you might end up looking kind of hot?

Flakes

You have flakes? You have fungus. It's naturally occurring (in fact, we all harbour it) and if you do get dandruff, your scalp is just overreacting to your fungus friend. This almost allergic reaction speeds up your natural skin cell turnover. It doesn't shed properly and finally leaves the scalp in clumpy flakes. Also, you might feel irritated and itchy. You should be able to fix flakes by using anti-dandruff

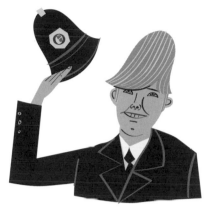

and – when you remove it later on – quickly restyle with damp (not wet) hands. Using water-soluble wax or light pomade means that you can refix easily later in the day.

Goop Slime

Goop slime is an overload of product that dribbles down your face as you go about your day. You leave home with perfectly styled high-gloss hair and end up looking like your face has been varnished hours later. The solution is to rein in your product use, try an oil-minimising lotion for your forehead, and steer clear of heavy pomades.

shampoo, but if it's still building up like a snowdrift, or if your flakes are yellowish and large, it's probably time for a visit to the doctor to get something a little stronger.

Hat Hair

This one is easy: don't wear hats. But if you must (maybe you're a policeman or a bishop) make sure your hair is completely dry before you put on your hat,

Hitting the Bottle

Men dye their hair for the same reason lots of women do – they're not ready to go grey yet (although their hair thinks otherwise). For them, the connotations of age are too closely bound to grey hair and they prefer what is perceived to be a more youthful look.

Unless you're incredibly skilled with home dyeing, and can guarantee you won't dye your forehead/ears/dog in the process, visit a professional. You can spot a bad DIY dye job a mile off: with grey roots showing, or bits you've over-dyed sticking out in clumps, this halfway house between grey and colour isn't where you want to be. But if you insist, apply dye to clean, damp hair; never deviate from the instructions, and make sure you've protected your sink or bathtub with old towels (whatever happens, rinsing out the colour will splash dye everywhere). Don't do it standing in the shower – unless you want a dyed back. And watch out for allergies –

most permanent and semi-permanent dyes insist on a patch test before using. This isn't overkill: hair-dye allergies are rare but can be severe.

Muppet Fluff

Fluffy with just a little touch of Muppet? Super-fine short hair can be tamed by tweaking your shampoo routine. Continue to rinse your hair daily with warm (not too hot) water, but only wash it occasionally. Natural hair oil will start to build up, giving your hair more body and texture; use a little conditioner on non-wash days to keep it all fresh-smelling.

Long, Crisp & Dry

Think about it: the longer your hair gets – and the further from your scalp – the dryer it becomes. Natural hair oils are the best remedy for keeping moisture intact, so actually washing less might be the answer. Do you have long hair that's dry at the ends? Try skipping the occasional wash, or switch to a milder shampoo that won't strip out all those nourishing oils. You can also try a little gents' hair powder (or dry shampoo) to freshen up your scalp if it gets too oily during this changeover period.

Tried & Tested: Silver Foxery

I've tried and tested being grey, but not really by choice. When I discovered my first grey hair at the age of 19 or so I wasn't too surprised. My dad – who's been almost completely grey since I've known him – maintains he had a grey streak at the age of 16 (but that might just be a Dad legend based on no truth whatsoever). I've never thought it makes me look old – or worried much about it – but sometimes I do wonder what I would look like with silver-free hair. There are cuts and treatments that make it look good (being without pigment, grey hair is hollow and can therefore be a little dryer than dark hair), and growing it very long does sometimes look a little witchy in the wrong light. But keeping it slick and well cared for means that it looks – in my humble opinion – pretty good. I might not be in the running for the Silver Fox of the Year award (not an actual thing), but if there was a Silver Squirrel or Weasel accolade, I would totally nail it.

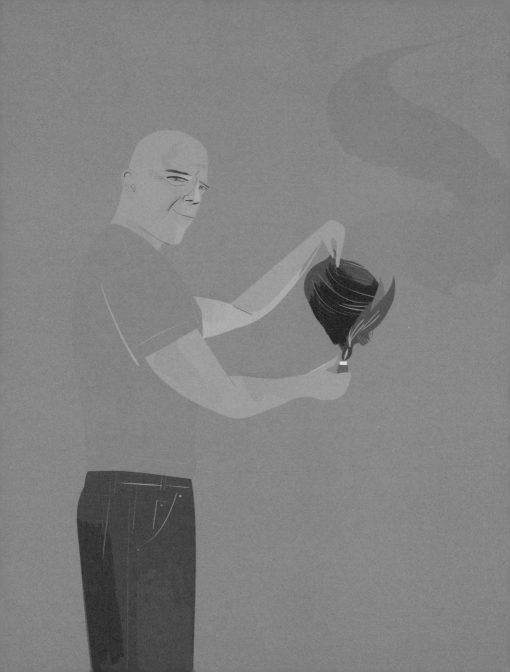

How to Be Bald

This is all about confidence and self-acceptance. And exfoliating. And accepting Bruce Willis as your personal saviour. Like progress, you can't usually stop the balding process, but for most of us it's a slow creep rather than a shock fallout. Most men have receded a little by their early 20s although this isn't always a precursor to balding – if it's in your genes it'll happen. The drugs do work, but they are not that effective if you start using them too late. Before BD (Bald Day, the moment you clipper or shave off your remaining hair), continue to visit the barber; a bit of expert clippering can work wonders with your look. Wash regularly with a mild moisturising face wash – or even a tiny amount of shampoo (an anti-dandruff or dry-scalp shampoo will help with itching); exfoliate once a week; apply moisturiser with sunblock. Pay your scalp the attention you would give your face and watch out for an over-oily appearance. You can counter this with bald-head wipes (yes, such things exist) or an oil-minimising moisturiser. If you're bald by choice and love to shave right down to the skin, exfoliating is a must. Avoid the comb-over and experiment with facial hair if you feel like changing up your look. Remember, you're Bruce Willis.

TREATMENTS & TECH

Cosmetic Hair-Loss Treatments

There is, of course, a sciencey reason for male pattern baldness: it's the creation of a hormone that, when its levels increase, has a sort of Godzilla effect on naturally occurring testosterone, turning it into dihydrotestosterone (DHT). High amounts of DHT cause your hair follicles to produce weaker hairs until they die out entirely. Bye-bye, barnet. Medications can help: Regaine (known as Rogaine in the US) is an over-the-counter lotion you apply twice a day. Most people find it effective, although it wears off as soon as you stop applying. Propecia is an oral treatment that also has a healthy success rate.

Surgical-Hair Loss Options

The hair follicles on the back and sides of your head usually happily pump out hair all your days, regardless of what's going on up top, so surgeons remove follicular units from these areas, via a process known as follicular unit extraction (FUE), slice these up into tiny chunks or thin strips, and graft them onto your bald bits via tiny incisions. The donor site (usually your head, but hair from your beard and body can also be considered) is closed with stitches and is usually hidden by your hair. You'll most likely need a few sessions to achieve a full head of hair, but the grafted follicles will be added in stages so the grow-back (once healed) should look pretty natural. Bruising (sometimes around the eyes) and a bit of scabbing can occur, plus potential itchiness – and you'll be back on the slab (or in a chair, rather) every two to four months before completion. FUE can also be used to restore or transform eyebrows and eyelashes. A scalp reduction procedure is also an option – where a segment of tissue is removed like orange peel, bringing your hairline back down to pre-baldness levels.

There's a school of thought that surgical hair-loss treatments for young men should be avoided, as transplanted hair follicles might be programmed to expire in years to come. Around 30 years old and up is preferable.

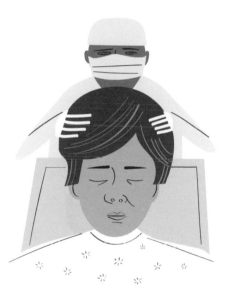

Icons of Grooming

MR DAVID LYNCH

Lofty, handsome and impossibly weird, David Lynch is much more than the lauded film director who lays bare the oddities of small-town life; he's an artist, musician, coffee-bean peddler and silent-nightclub designer. His trademark look – black suit and simple white shirt – is topped off with a silvery grey peak of wonderfully wavy hair.

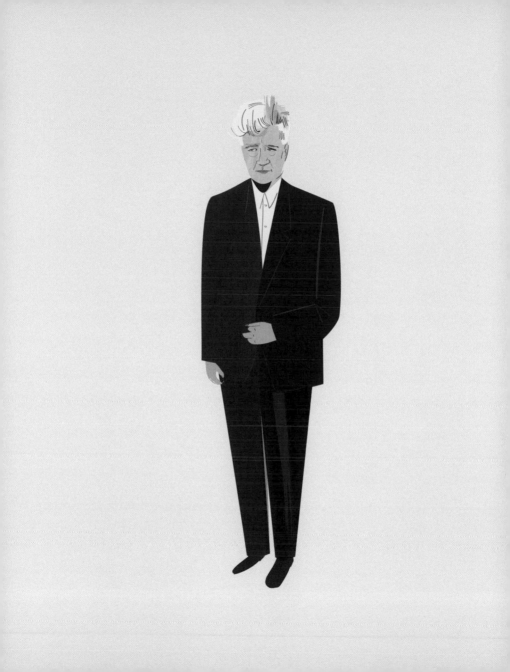

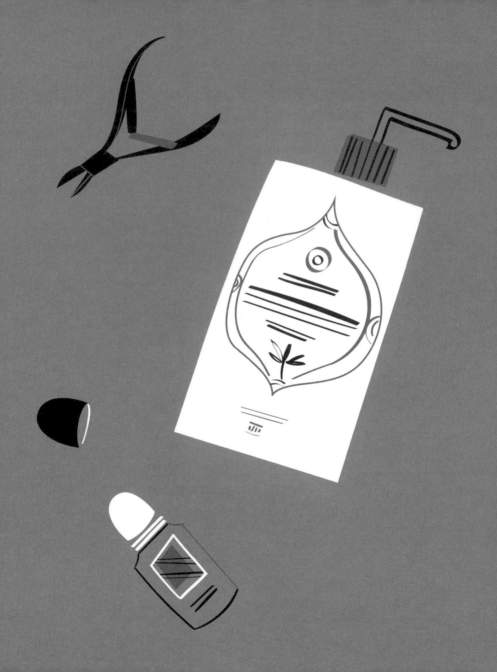

Chapter Four

The
Body

Perhaps not the most refined science but fitness and wellness experts identify just three main male body types – ectomorph, endomorph and mesomorph. These are techy terms, devised by the late American psychologist W. H. Sheldon for: lean and long, more to love or well built with a near-magical tendency to gain muscle. Whatever your body shape, it pays to keep it clean, clippered and smelling good.

KNOW YOUR BODY TYPE

You can be anywhere on the body-type matrix, sharing attributes from more than one of the categories. Ectomorphs tend to stay skinny despite hours in the gym, endomorphs struggle to shift their swerves and curves, and mesomorphs... well, have you seen the size of their guns?

LEAN AND LONG

You're long with gangly limbs and knobbly elbows – like a marathon runner. You're an ectomorph. Good news: your metabolism is set to light-speed. Bad news: you'll find it very hard to bulk up. A diet high in calories, carbs, fat and protein might help with muscle gain.

MORE TO LOVE

You're prone to roundness. Round head, round body, and short-ish limbs. And you're also prone to flab. You're an endomorph. Your body loves fat like a fat person loves cake. According to Sheldon, you're always this way – even if you work out, eat well and are super-toned with mega-pecs, you'll still have the tendency to put on weight when you so much as look at an enchilada.

THE GUNSHOW

Well, look at you, mesomorph. You're pretty lean, muscular and strong. Everything's in proportion; you have wide shoulders with an efficient metabolism that makes it easy to lose fat, and building new muscle takes little effort. People (like me) are jealous of you. And you probably love it.

Knowing your predisposition to a certain body type can be liberating: been working out for years but can't seem to build muscle on your spindly limbs? Or do you feel as though you eat

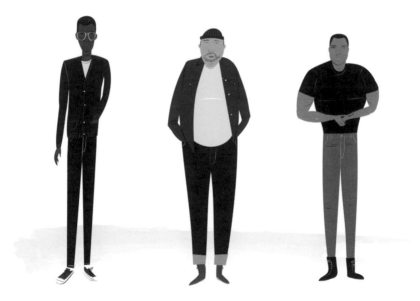

just as much string cheese as your friend but it's you that puts on weight and not them? Knowing where you stand on Sheldon's morph matrix can help guide you with your exercise choices and cake intake. Oh, to be a mesomorph...

YOUR GROOMING ROUTINE

HOW TO WASH

I usually think of my dad as a good, solid yardstick for the average man's approach to grooming: he has never used moisturiser or sunblock, he always asks for an All Over cut, and – I'm pretty sure – he washes with shampoo rather than soap or shower gel. (I know this because the only thing I ever find in his bathroom is the supermarket own-brand anti-dandruff shampoo, and any grooming product I buy him as a gift is gratefully received but lurks untouched in a cupboard somewhere.) Thing is, there's not a huge difference between shampoo and shower gel. Designed to remove oil from your hair, shampoo might

How to Get a Great Set of Guns

The Golden Fleece of men's fitness; whole industries are devoted to the male obsession with growing a plump, meaty set of biceps (and it has to be said, they look pretty awesome). There are powders and potions, super-charged supplements and left-field fitness programmes and diets, but biceps really only respond to one thing: weight training. Heaving impossibly heavy weights in the gym creates tiny tears in your muscles that your body fixes, overcompensating in anticipation of you doing it again. Your muscles slowly grow bigger (not actually in the gym – muscle forms when you're at rest) and your weights have to get steadily weightier the bigger you'd like to be. Perform big lifts as well as bicep curls to put extra stress on your body and encourage even more muscle build-up. Experiment with different grips, take your time (follow the 'one second up, three seconds down' rule) and pump away until you can pump no more. Finally, with a few dumbbell kickbacks, work up your triceps, the often forgotten muscle that sits on the back of your upper arm: this will lift up your biceps, making your arms look huge – like you've taped hunks of meatloaf to them.

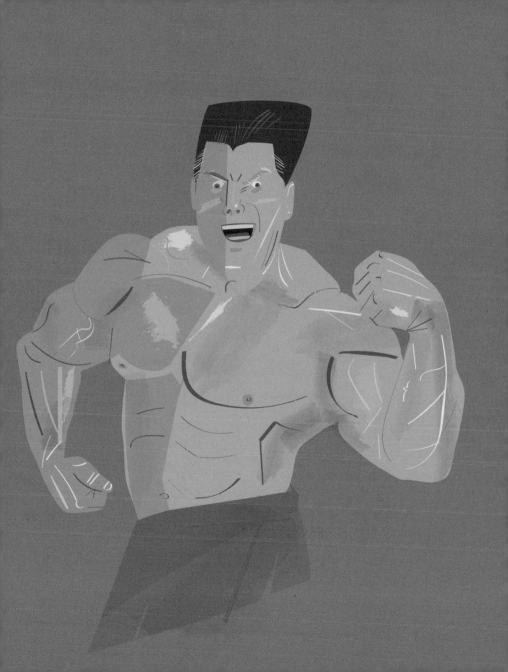

dry your skin a little, but it still does the job. With washing, it doesn't really matter how you get there – just as long as you do. Where you shouldn't skimp is the dry-off afterwards: wet and warm is just how the bacteria and fungus on your skin like it – so it's important to dry all those, um, cracks and crevices: between your toes, inside your ears... Washing without drying properly is like treating your fungus friends to a spa day.

BODY MOISTURISING

At the very least, moisturise with a body lotion at least once a week. If you're playing lots of sports or working out lots – and are showering more than usual – increase your applications to once a day. Your face gets all the benefits of moisturiser, why shouldn't your body? Apply after a shower – when you've dried off but your skin is slightly damp – to seal in moisture. Prepping your body first with a body exfoliator will aid absorption.

DRY SKIN BRUSHING

Crusty elbows, scaly knees and bumpy arms can be sanded off via dry brushing – the invigorating exfoliation technique that is perfect for sensitive skin. Using a natural bristle brush, brush your body in long sweeping strokes starting with your limbs, then torso, always moving towards your heart. You'll be sweeping away dead skin cells, promoting circulation, and buffing your skin to smoothness. Invest in a soft natural bristle brush (buy one specifically for skin brushing – i.e. not from the hardware store) and get grooming just before you jump in the shower. Dry off as normal and apply a body moisturiser. Every two to three days should be enough – and you should notice a difference in a week or two.

EPSOM SALTS

It is the cheap, affordable grooming cure-all that does real wonders for your skin and hair, and is said to be a hangover remedy, all in one. Epsom salt, otherwise known as magnesium sulfate, can even clean your tiles, deter slugs and keep your lawn green. For human usage, about two cups of salts should do it, added to a super-hot bath (preferably after dry skin brushing) where you should soak for around 20 minutes. It is thought that magnesium and sulfate can both be easily absorbed through the skin, each with its own benefits – from stress relief to softening skin. Don't try it if you have circulatory problems – it's pretty stimulating – and be careful as you step out of the bath: you might feel a little woozy. Have a room-temp shower afterwards to cool off.

HAIRY BITS

Remember the air-punch when you discovered your first hair down there? And again when more turned up to join the party? But for some of us, the process of growing body hair just didn't stop and, as an adult, we're more shag pile than shaggable. Some remove pubic hair for hygiene reasons; or perhaps you have a personal preference to thin it out a bit, give it a little shape – like a flat top, or teased into an afro? Or maybe you like it removed completely: ripped off at the waxer's, or discreetly clippered at home?

Here's how to do it:

Waxing

It sounds horrific. Heated wax is spread with a spatula over your hairiest bits before a therapist uses a strip to remove the wax along with the hair. The torturous-sounding treatment is tempered by the professionalism and skill of your therapist, and it is so quick that it's more than possible to grin and bear it. In minutes you're left with super-soft and smooth skin that feels clean and cool – and it certainly allows for more pronounced muscle defin-ition. Sensitive skin can react strongly, and a post-session exfoliation is essential. Having regular treatments is beneficial as it usually makes the process easier and speedier as hair can grow back a little finer each time.

Laser

Prepare to have your intimate areas zapped. Via medical laser, hair can be removed from almost any area of your body – with the laser beam heating and permanently destroying hair follicles in all the wrong places. It is not cheap and you usually need a course of treatments – and sometimes there's an odd sort of BBQ aroma that makes you feel hungry for ribs (until you realise what it is).

Sugaring

A heated sugar paste is applied to your hairy areas and removed by a therapist, either by hand or with cloth strips. It's said to be less

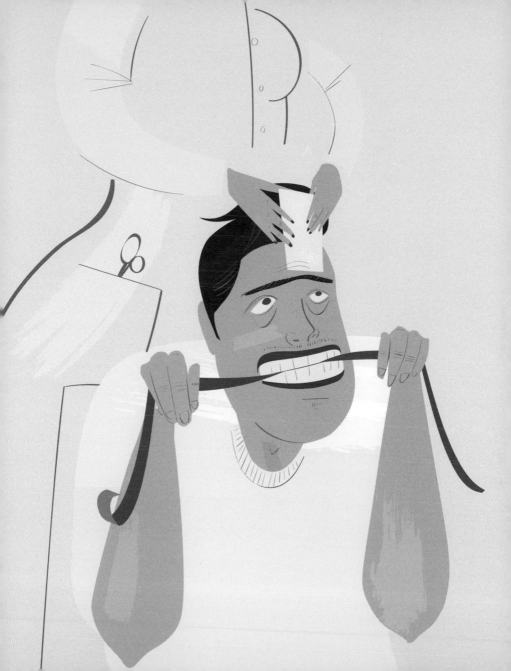

painful than waxing, with less potential for allergic reaction, as it is 100 per cent natural. Exfoliation is essential to prevent ingrown hairs – use a simple exfoliator or a rough washcloth.

Clippering

This is the DIY job you probably shouldn't call your dad for advice on. Clippering at home is cheap and effective – but it's easy to make a mistake or be a little overzealous. Trim too short and you are left with spiky hair that will feel itchy and uncomfortable. And watch out for nicks and cuts. This option is best for men who are moderately hairy, have a steady hand and know when enough is enough. Also, use a clipper specifically for body hair.

Shaving

The same rules apply as when you shave your face: make sure that whatever you are shaving is clean and prepped, the hair is post-shower soft, and you're using a shaving oil or fine cream so that you can see what you're doing. Post-shave exfoliation is essential to avoid ingrown hairs. Be prepared for bristly grow-back (and crazy itching when this occurs) and the amount of time needed to keep it in tiptop condition. It's a commitment – but they're your balls.

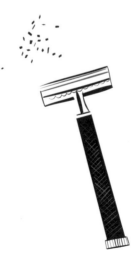

TROUBLESOME PROBLEMS

WEIRD SMELLS

You stink? Here's how to fix it. First and foremost, up your hygiene – and not just showering, but drying off properly and keeping your clothes super-clean and fresh. Avoid wearing man-made fibres (this includes cotton-poly mix fabrics) that don't allow your skin to breathe, make you sweat and retain bad odours that seep out after a couple of hours of wear. Next, check your sweat levels. It's natural to perspire – it's the body doing what it should – but if you think you're sweating excessively you should see if a doctor can help. And eat well: toning down stinkier herbs and spices will help, as well as cutting down your sugar and caffeine intake.

BACKNE

Treating acne on your back is much the same as how you might treat it on your face. A salt bath can help kill off bacteria and fungus, help dry out pimples, and – if it's mild acne – exfoliating (use a loofah or scrubbing brush) can help, too.

How to Shave Your Balls

Why the obsession with ball-shaving? Why do we hate that sparse hair that covers our plums so much that it needs to be whipped off with a razor to reveal a shiny smooth set underneath? Shaving down there is a real commitment: it's not for the slapdash or short on time. The spiky grow-back is itchy, uncomfortable and a little dangerous, too – should we really be playing about in our nether regions with a razor? If you're hellbent on the porn-star look, there are a few things to consider. Start off with a body-hair trimmer to shorten hair prior to shaving, and use a brand-new, high-quality, super-sharp safety razor. Make sure your hair and skin are clean, soft and supple; shaving post-bath is ideal (but splash a little cold water down there to tighten the skin). Use a good-quality shaving cream or oil and, with a surgeon's precision, start to slowly shave away. Rinse halfway through to admire your handiwork and highlight any bits you've missed, and finish off with the application of a cooling post-shave balm. Aftercare is essential – you must use an exfoliator. And there you have it: a set of balls as shiny and clean looking as a couple of freshly boiled eggs.

The Body

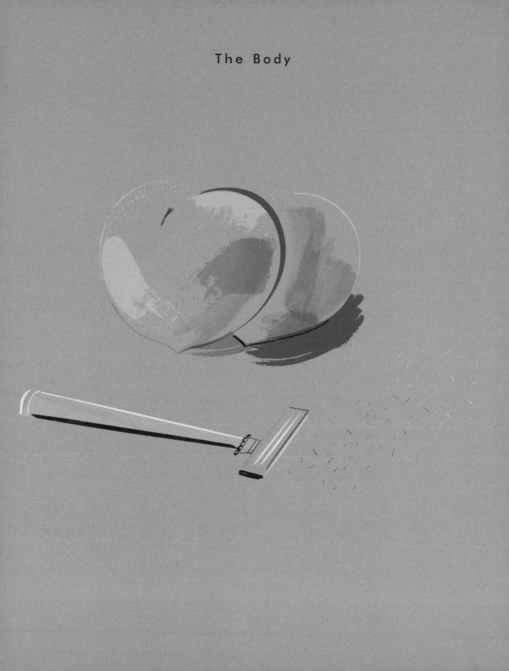

TREATMENTS & TECH

Full Body Exfoliation

It's tricky – and mildly mind-numbing – exfoliating your whole body yourself. What about that tricky upper-middle back part? So, why not pay someone else to do it? Book in for a whole body exfoliation every couple of months at your local spa (or once a month if you are extra-scaly). You'll be moisturised afterwards and achieve an impossibly velvety-all-over finish, guaranteed.

Spray Tanning

Although a little sun exposure is essential for your body to absorb vitamin D, don't ever use a sunbed. Just don't. Think of them as slightly greasy skin time machines that will transport your epidermis to 2056 in minutes. Instead, fake a beach body with artisanal spray tanning: the freehand application of tanning dye to accentuate muscle defin-ition. At a grooming salon, skilled therapists can spray on a six-pack and more using layers of tanning mist. It's less techy treatment, more trompe l'oeil on your droopy bits. The traditional all-over treat-ment is effective too – but if you have extremely light skin, it's rarely going to look completely natural, so it's best to go to an expert. Less really is more.

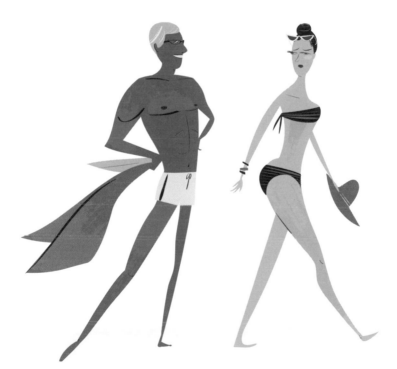

FINGERS & FEET

If the eyes are the windows of the soul, hands are the trapdoor to the psyche. Gnarled, dry hands, with BBQ-sauce-encrusted fingernails are a sure sign of a careless mind – so it pays to keep them up.

I once perched nervously on the edge of an Eames chair sweating my way through a super-tough job interview – one of those situations so intense that afterwards you are haunted by tiny details – and I have always remembered my interviewer's nails. He was the head of an international luxury men's outfitters that turns over millions each year – and worked seven days a week flying all over the world –

plus was a full-time dad to three kids. And his nails? Impeccable. Clipped short (not stumpy), buffed to a high shine – they were the executive nails of a man at the top of his game. I didn't get the job, but I remember thinking I should at least have a manicure like him; that the super-successful of this world had clawed their way up out of the gutter with perfectly buffed nails. I didn't get a chance to see his feet, but I'm pretty sure they would've looked fairly buffed, too.

The Manicure

You'll need clippers, a nail file and buffer, plus some hand lotion or coconut oil to finish. First up, wash your hands and use clippers to cut nails short (but not stumpy), and round off the edges with a nail file (moving in one direction only). Then use the buffer – starting with the coarsest side then gradating up to the smoothest, wiping away dust as you go. Wipe your nails clean and apply coconut oil (or just hand lotion) to your cuticles (the tiny section of dry skin that connects to your nail) to keep them soft. Congratulations, you now have executive nails!

The Pedicure

Much the same as a manicure, but you'll need the flexible spine of a youthful man. You'll need toenail clippers, a nail file and buffer, and, again, some hand lotion or coconut oil to finish. First up, wash your feet thoroughly and dry between your toes, looking out for any broken skin that might be the sign of athlete's foot. Using tweezers, gently pick out any debris from the sides of the nails – usually sock-related fluff – and then use clippers to cut your nails short, in a straight, horizontal line. Use a nail file to round off the edges that might otherwise encourage all sorts of problems, including ingrowing nails. Then use the buffer – starting with the coarsest side then gradating up to the smoothest, wiping away dust as you go. Wipe your nails clean and apply coconut oil (or just lotion) to your cuticles to keep them soft.

Troublesome Mani/Pedi Problems

HANGNAILS

The devil's work. Hangnails are the dry, brittle, triangular-shaped flaps of skin that appear around your fingernails and you absent-mindedly tear off. They are painful and don't look great. Hangnails are usually the result of dehydration caused by cold weather, harsh chemicals or repeated washing. Regular nail maintenance really helps prevent them, but if you already have one throbbing away on one of your digits, soften it in warm water for a few minutes, then snip it off with a pair of clippers, and add a little bacterial lotion until it heals.

SWEATY HANDS

If you feel your hands or feet are too sweaty there are a few clever hacks that will get you through clammier times. Hands: keep them clean, use an alcohol-based hand sanitiser (that will help the sweat evaporate), use an antiperspirant on your palms, and always carry some tissues to dry off with before you shake hands with people. But if you feel it is too severe, talk to your doctor – sweaty hands are usually quite easy to fix. Botox is occasionally an option with really strong results.

FEET DE FROMAGE

Feet: they're naturally sweaty. In fact, they pump out around a cup of sweat a day, producing more per square inch than anywhere else on your body. This high concentration of sweat, plus naturally occurring fungus and bacteria – coupled with a nice, warm and damp environment inside your socks – means your feet can stink like an artisan cheese platter. Different types of naturally occurring bacteria on your body let off different smells, so there's a panoply of aromas your feet can produce. Getting rid of foot odour means tackling sweat, bacteria and fungus. Wear shoes and socks made of natural materials, dab a little surgical spirit between your toes, use medicated insoles and keep your feet clean and dry.

Tried & Tested: The Medi-Pedi

Margaret Dabbs has what most might think is an odd claim to fame: she is arguably the world's best (and definitely the most in demand) cosmetic foot specialist. Based in London, she has a fiercely loyal clientele of men and women – some of whom regularly fly across the globe to get their feet done by the expert herself.

Her Medical Pedicure is the full works – a 45-minute treatment performed on a dry foot to ensure long-lasting results. There's the removal of all dead and dry skin, nails are shaped, buffed and moisturised, and the feet are left revitalised. In fact, people say they often look 'ten years younger'. She worked wonders on mine and dispelled any nervousness on my part – when I took off my socks and unleashed my monkey claws on her – with real enthusiasm for her job. For weeks afterwards I had feet I wasn't ashamed to get out on the beach.

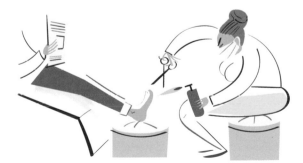

Icons of Grooming

MR TONY WARD

Californian-born model, actor, artist and designer (among other things), Tony Ward has been the focus of fashion and style imagery for decades. His famous debut in his undies in the 1980s as a Calvin Klein model with images by Herb Ritts was upstaged in the 1990s when he became Madonna's boyfriend. His approach to style – laid-back, fresh and a little bit grungy (he has more than 20 excellent tattoos) – has earned him a sort of anti-model status. And he's a fan of Grandpa's Wonder Pine Tar Soap.

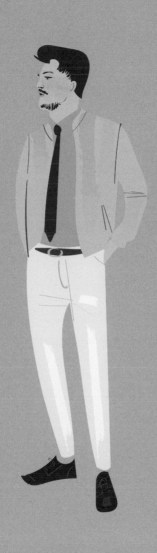

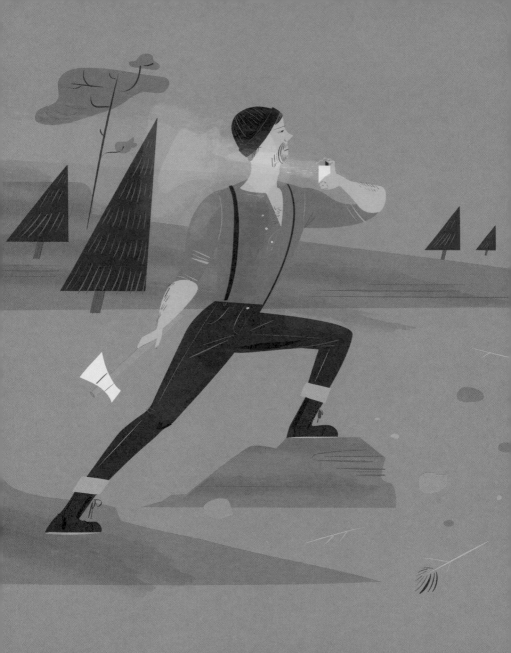

How to Find the Perfect Fragrance

Different fragrances conjure memories, thoughts and feelings, and mixed well they can be emotionally charged. You can use the seasons to guide your choices, sticking to a bright citrus in the summer, and rich, woody notes in the winter – and build up three or four fragrances you love. Eau de parfum is the strongest, containing up to 15 per cent pure, super-strong fragrance – a potent blend that lingers on your skin (great for winter); eau de toilette is next, at around 9 per cent. Eau de cologne contains anything up to 5 per cent fragrance (good in summer), and aftershave has no more than 3 per cent (and is probably not worth investing in). Spray on a high-quality fragrance and its top notes will hit you right away – usually a fresh, sharp aroma that gives way to the middle notes, the heart of the scent. The bass notes appear last – usually deep and musky – and linger the longest. Apply to your chest and back before you put on your clothes to let the aroma slowly seep out, or spritz a little inside your jacket. And now you stink: in a good way.

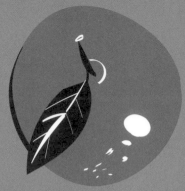

Chapter Five
Wellness

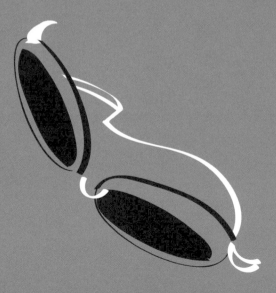

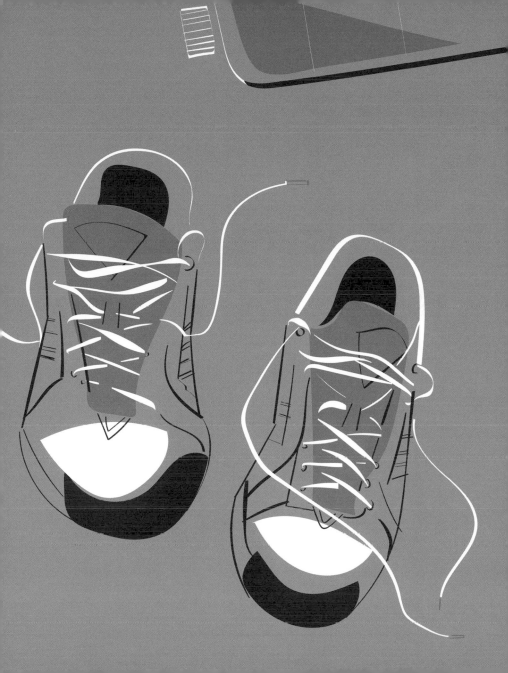

Wellness: the contemporary term that sounds more dreamcatcher and scented candle than hardcore weights and protein shakes. But it's a nifty term that encompasses fitness and health with long-term life changes, a bit of ball-feeling and a little mindfulness on the side. Meditation is a hugely effective treatment for stress, anxiety, lack of focus, relationship problems, addictive behaviour and more. Put in the effort and you'll get back peace of mind and a sense of wellbeing, real focus and creativity, and better relationships. Forealsies.

FITNESS

Wild Swimming

Swimming in cold-water rivers and lakes can activate your immune system, burn calories and leave you feeling amazing – but is the latter a fitness response or just sheer relief in having survived the session? Swimming is great for aerobic fitness; you will lose fat and increase muscle. But icy water is a bit of a risk for some: a sudden drop in temperature puts huge strain on the heart. Best to build up your tolerance with quick dips.

Pilates

There are different types of Pilates, but the tenets are the same: the system of stretching and maintaining tricky postures borrows from yoga and martial arts. It's great for strengthening muscles that support the spine, helping those with back problems. It works by strengthening your core muscles – namely, the abdominals – and the series of stretches can make good posture more achievable, as you become more aware of your body. Pilates' slow pace belies super-powers in building muscle, especially around the stomach and upper body.

Running

The multimillion-dollar running industry is heavily promoted by sports apparel makers and underlined by a booming economy of international marathons and urban running crews. Marathon training pushes people to the max; there are even ultramarathons and mud-splattered iron man triathlons, and training for them leaves you extremely lean and fit. Running won't increase muscle size (it makes muscle more efficient, not bigger), but you'll lose weight and really increase your aerobic capacity. Remember to super-power your run with sprint intervals.

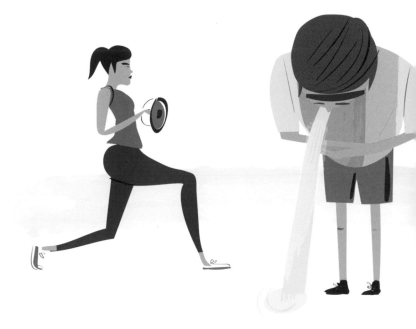

HIIT

Want to get ripped but can't be bothered putting in the time? If you don't mind throwing up mid-class, then HIIT is for you. High-intensity interval training is the nifty idea to alternate 30-second bursts of intense aerobic exercise with slower recovery periods where you're jogging lightly on a treadmill listening to Taylor Swift on your headphones. HIIT is claimed to have the same benefits as undertaking normal exercise (such as running or cycling) for far longer. And by some miracle, it works, and it even seems to lessen your appetite (you don't

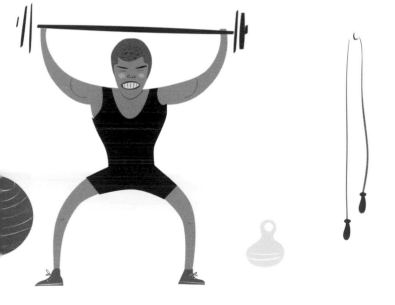

necessarily get that starved feeling that is common after you have been swimming, say). For instance, a ten-minute fast-but-not-furious cycle ride with two 20-second super-fast I'm-going-to-throw-up sprints is about the same as a solid 45 minutes in the saddle. HIIT puts a real strain on your body and heart so it should only be undertaken by the fit and healthy.

CrossFit

The cultish fitness phenomenon that is the angry little brother to SoulCycle. Ostensibly, CrossFit is an extreme circuit-training class where you perform everyday functional movements and lift heavy loads competitively with other nervous-looking guys. Your presence is required the following weeks to chart your improvement, and the tough environment, competitive element and intense

weights get real results: namely, a drop in body fat and increase in aerobic capacity, and an overarching sense of smugness when describing what you did to your friends. Drawbacks are both the cost – sessions are usually expensive – and the potential risk of injury.

Tried & Tested: Tempo Pilates

Pilates, the system of stretching, weights and tricky posture exercises, can be performed on a mildly cheesy yoga mat – or on a reformer bed. Tempo Pilates – devised by industry celeb Daniel Le Roux – is a special routine on a reformer bed set to up-tempo music. Like a rowing machine, the bed can slide horizontally with pulleys with hoops at the end to which springs are attached that vary the weight – and therefore the resistance. Trying out a class in London, it turns out you can lie on the bed, kneel, stand or squat at the edge of it to work different muscle groups. And you can add free weights to work your arms. There's even a curious rubber-ended pole at one point, and a plastic ring like a bike wheel you can try to break between your knees. Starting the class lying down is brilliant but little indication of the horrors of what's to come – and a position that feels easy develops in just a few seconds into something that makes your muscles burn. It's intense, so you can achieve real greatness very quickly. Excellent for back pain, jelly belly, and general flexibility. Within a few weeks my core was so strong I could pick something up off the floor – without groaning.

———

DIET

Paleo

Paleo, the fitness industry's current diet obsession, takes inspiration from ancient hunter-gatherers and according to Paleo obsessives, is the way humans are actually supposed to eat. This seems to resonate with those who see string cheese or chicken nuggets as a

Man Made

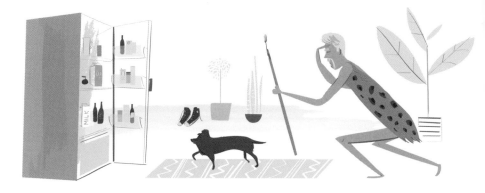

food crime and seek a better, more balanced way of eating. Evolutionary medicine man Loren Cordain's 2002 book, *The Paleo Diet*, is considered the seminal guide on the subject. Since then, all manner of Paleo diets and guides have been drawn up, but they're all based on a few common principles: you're encouraged to pile on the protein, seeking out grass-fed and wild varieties while avoiding corn- or grain-fed animals, and dried and cured processed meats. In fact, grains are out completely – which includes pasta, bread, rice, even cake – and legumes (lentils, peas, beans) are also a no-no. Finally, dairy is allowed but in tiny quantities, but you're encouraged to eat naturally occurring fat – from meat, fish or avocados and nuts, especially coconut.

The 5:2

Unbelievably simple – and effective – this eating plan is based around five days of normal eating and then, two days a week, you reduce your calorie intake to 600 calories (500 for women). You control which days you battle through with little more than a stock cube and a banana – and you're free to eat whatever the hell you like the other five days. It works. Over weeks, you lose weight to a point where you can reduce or stop your fast days altogether. Generally, you don't binge-eat tacos on your normal-eating days as your appetite diminishes a little, along with your weight.

Tried & Tested: The Whole30

Dallas and Melissa Hartwig's bestselling book, *It Starts With*

Food, attempts to shift us away from addictive, processed, sugar-rich Frankenfoods and on to something altogether more healthy, for just 30 days. The idea is that a month of eating healthy wholefoods will be long enough to break bad habits, 'starve the sugar dragon' and transform your body. It's not a weight-loss diet (but almost all W30 devotees lose weight by the end of it) and is concerned with the inflammatory effects of certain foodstuffs, challenging you to see how you might feel without them. It's tough. Dallas and Melissa are extremely strict and any major slip-ups will send you right back to Day 1. But it gets easier and the food is great – grass-fed or wild meat and fish, eggs, loads of vegetables, a little fruit, and fat – three times a day. Snacking is frowned upon. But that's it – no sugar, alcohol, grains or beans – just healthy

How to Make the Perfect Green Smoothie

And it doesn't contain kale. David Frenkiel and Luise Vindahl are Swedish and Danish respectively and experts in amazing-looking and -tasting vegetarian food. Their *Green Kitchen Stories* blog and two recipe books are pretty much the go-to for anyone wanting to eat and drink healthily and happily. Their Green Recovery Smoothie is the best out there – and ridiculously easy to make.

GREEN RECOVERY SMOOTHIE

Celery and banana are rich in the electrolytes sodium and potassium (which you lose when you sweat). Together with the proteins in the hemp powder and nut butter, they are the perfect ingredients in a recovery drink. Keep hydrated and drink this Green Recovery Smoothie after a workout for best results: ◆ 1 celery stalk with leaves ◆ 1 ripe banana, peeled ◆ 1 kiwi, peeled ◆ ½ avocado, stoned ◆ juice of 1 lime ◆ 1 tbsp hemp protein powder (optional) ◆ 1 tbsp almond butter or soaked almonds ◆ 1 cup (240 ml) coconut water or plant milk of your choice. ◆ Mix all the ingredients in a blender with a few ice cubes until smooth.

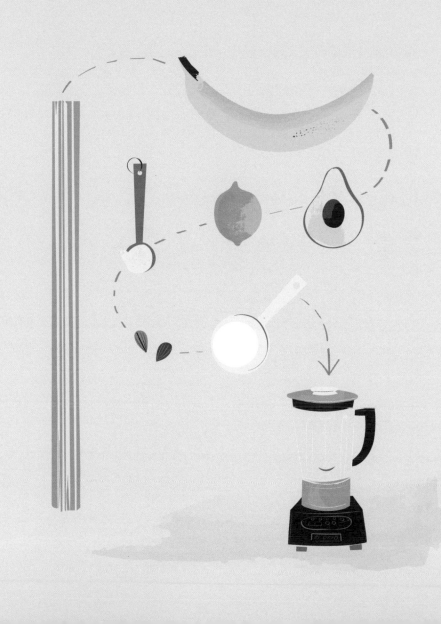

wholefoods. In one month I'd eaten more than ever – including a ridiculous amount of eggs and sweet potato – but by the end I felt super-calm, smug, and was waking early full of intense energy (the Hartwigs refer to this feeling as 'tiger blood'). And – for the first time in years – my love handles had totally disappeared. For that, Dallas and Melissa, I love you.

ROUTINE MAINTENANCE

TEETH

British men aren't known for their good teeth. While a hygienic few brush, floss and gargle with gay abandon, it's the others who give us a bad name. Their diet of red wine, coffee and cigarettes can leave them with a smile like a row of wooden clothes pegs. Unfortunately for our teeth, and the self-esteem of dentists, we rarely consider having them looked at by a professional. Whether your teeth are like Tic Tacs or tombstones, it pays to look after them, whatever shape

Wellness

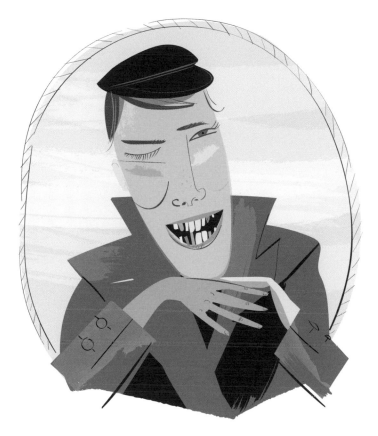

and state they're in. Keep them bright and white by cutting down sugar, caffeine and smoking. Fizzy drinks, even sugar-free ones, can destroy your teeth's enamel. Flossing is a must – it removes bits of food that get caught between teeth every time you eat, and really helps prevent gum disease (the main causes of tooth loss in adults). Facing a dentist's receptionist twice a year seems like a cross we all should bear. Unless you want all your teeth to fall out and be replaced with clothes pegs.

DOWN BELOW

All working okay down there? Nothing to report? Great. But if not, it's easy to get it all seen to. A low embarrassment threshold can be deadly – with men letting health worries go unchecked to the point where they're much worse than they might have been. Add to your grooming routine a monthly testicular self-examination. Examine each testicle with both hands, placing the index and middle fingers underneath, with the thumbs placed on top. Roll the testicle gently between the thumbs and fingers; you shouldn't feel any pain, and don't be alarmed if one testicle seems slightly larger than the other – that's normal. Find the epididymis (the spaghetti-like structure behind the testicle that collects and carries sperm) so you won't mistake it for something that shouldn't be there – and then cop a feel. Any lumps or bumps, changes in density or pain should be immediately looked at by a doctor. Potentially embarrassing, yes. But guess what? Doctors don't care. They want to see you as quickly and efficiently as possible. And chances are that – whatever you are flopping out in front of them – they have seen something weirder earlier that day.

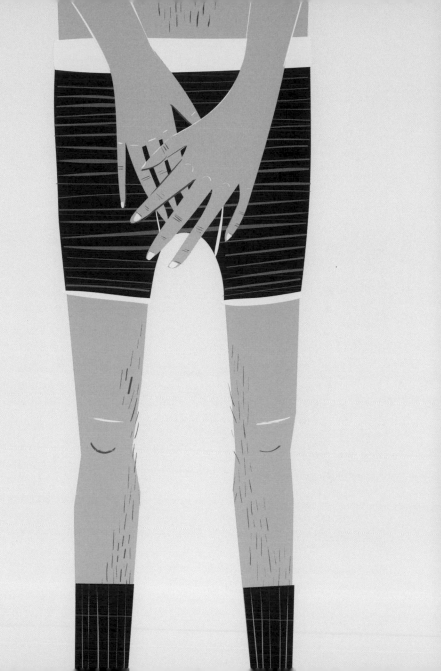

FEELING GOOD

Feeling Good

You've worked up your guns, eaten Paleo, felt up your balls – but what about your mind? Who's looking after that? There's shockingly little awareness of male mental health: society doesn't create a space for men to feel confident to talk openly about their stresses, thoughts and nagging self-critical feelings. If you're feeling stressed, anxious, or a bit down, what do you do?

Stress

Stress is designed to help us get out of physical danger. When we feel threatened, a part of our brain called the amygdala sets off an alarm bell that triggers the 'fight or flight' response of our nervous system, making us ready to respond. So we can move quickly, our blood is flooded with adrenaline and cortisol, increasing our heart rate and blood pressure. This means we can transport oxygen to our muscles quickly: perfect for when we were about to be ripped to shreds by a Velociraptor in olden times (okay, that was just in *Jurassic Park*), but it does little to help us in the modern world when we've missed the bus or forgotten to pick up the boss's lunch. Those high levels of adrenaline and cortisol play havoc with our bodies, shutting down non-essential systems, including our immune system. Constant stress eats away at your physical and mental wellbeing – it's a chemical imbalance, and ultimately needs to be dealt with.

Mindfulness & Meditation

Put out that incense immediately. This isn't about spirituality, this is about meditation: the taming of the mind and making real, science-based changes in your brain that make you feel... good. Mindfulness – the catch-all for the slowing down and focusing of your mental state – is a remedy for those everyday mental and emotional hurdles. If stress activates the fight-or-flight part of our nervous system,

meditation and mindfulness activate the other part of our nervous system – the calming, focused part.

When we meditate, our heart rate and breathing slows and our blood pressure drops. So, while activation of the fight-or-flight response can be damaging to the body and mind, meditating to achieve relaxation is restorative. Meditation – with all its spiritual and sometimes religious connotations – is the manly, scientific approach to better mental health. Some studies even suggest that in certain cases it is just as effective as anti-depressants. You can meditate by turning up the awareness of yourself and your surroundings: becoming aware of your body and physical sensations, and finally your thoughts; acknowledging them as neutrally as possible as they burst in and burst out of your

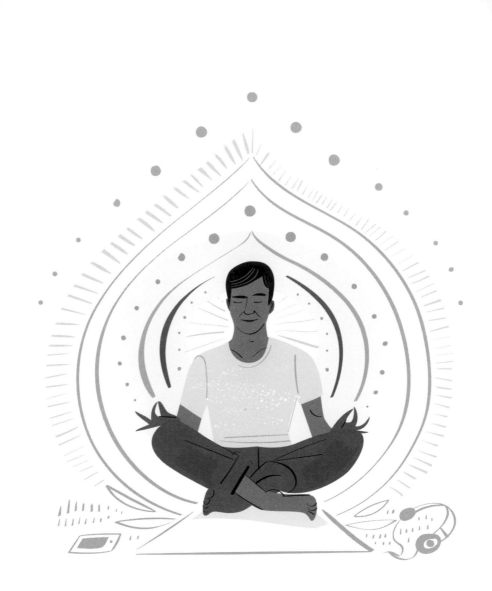

head; and then clearing your mind by focusing on breathing. Don't worry, it is not a fad. Humans have been doing it for more than 2,500 years, but it's easiest in a group session or on your headphones via an app (HeadSpace is great).

Feeling anxious and aren't able to indulge in an eight-week course of meditation? There's a hack to get there fast. Focus on one of your senses. Listen: become aware of background noise, really try to hear everything, all the fuzz and detail, and don't try to make sense of it. You'll be forcing your brain out of its fight-or-flight mode and into its more relaxed, thoughtful mode. And relax...

Depression

What can you do for a friend who's not feeling so great? Be good to them. Do they keep bouncing your calls? Keep calling them. Do they act a bit like an asshole? Be nice to them. There could be something else going on – so be their friend. And what to do if you yourself feel depressed? It's absolutley normal to feel down or anxious sometimes – most of us will experience it at some point in our lives – but you must ask for help. Remember, we live in a culture where men are prevented from having the confidence to seek help easily, but being quiet about how you feel isn't being strong. If you've hit a wall for whatever reason and just need to talk to someone, do it. Talk to a professional therapist.

In the meantime, be kind to yourself. That includes getting lots of sleep, exercise, and no booze. Remember that it will get better. Oh, and do see that professional. It might be your own doctor, or someone at the end of a phone line, But talk to someone.

Icons of Grooming

MR KARL-EDWIN GUERRE

NYC-based street-style photographer Karl-Edwin Guerre is the purveyor of the 'casual fly' look – a rounded style that often involves natty suiting, bold colour, painstaking attention to detail and some killer headgear. He believes it takes time to settle into your personal look; it's best not to push it. His own trajectory – from hip-hoppery and baggy clothes to slick, Wall Street look to laid-back and louche (with a touch of Willy Wonka) – is pretty impressive.

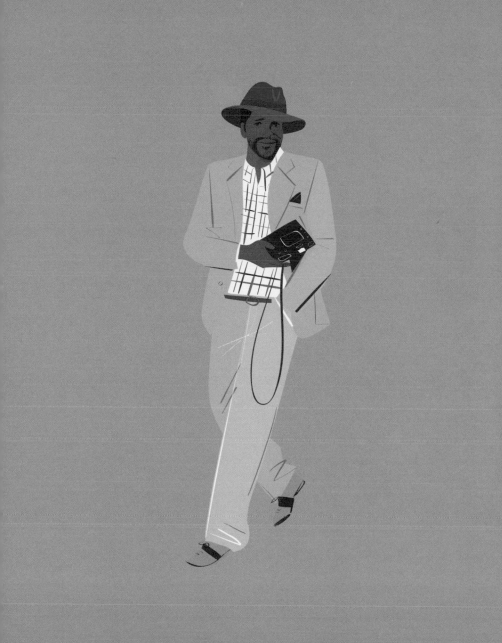

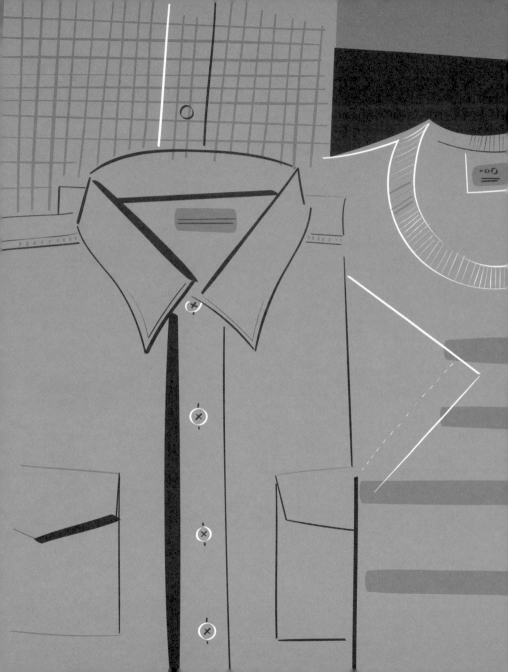

Chapter Six

Style

A pristine Savile Row suit, a battered and bashed-up Lewis Leathers biker jacket or baggy sweatpants covered in dog hair: what you wear is a projection of who you are. When you get dressed in the morning, you make a conscious (and unconscious) decision about what you communicate to the world. It's a visual representation of your personality, full of subtle codes and signs as to what sort of person you purport to be. It's how you pick out clothes in a store, or the hand-me-downs you treasure, and how you decide what not to wear – the hand-knitted 1980s batwing jumper you throw out, along with the fluoro tanga high-cut swimming briefs your grandma gave you for Christmas (speaking from experience). So, when men claim that they have no interest in clothes, and the jeans and T-shirt they are wearing are merely the first thing they found that was semi-clean this morning, it's just not true. Despite what men's mags would have you believe, there are no rules of how to dress. You can wear whatever you like. But so much of what we do – at work, out with friends – relies on an awareness of social convention if things are to go smoothly. It is like wearing a latex fetish-inspired onesie to the office, or a voluminous white lacy dress at a wedding (when you're not the bride). It's going to be awkward. The fail-safe approach – one that wins every time – is to balance fitting in (to be respectful) with sticking out (being yourself).

WHAT TO WEAR

Build a wardrobe of easy pieces that are simple and versatile, that you can wear to almost anywhere – from the office to the pub – with minor tweaks and tune-ups.

Navy blue or charcoal grey are the classics – black is a bit funereal, but also doable. The fit should be impeccable. Get really good advice here – you're looking for perfection.

The Suit

Weddings, funerals, bar mitzvahs... A proper suit should really work for its money, and be just as suitable for upscale events as it would a job interview or court appearance. To be truly versatile, you should pick something simple and understated: single-breasted, with little or no pattern, two buttons and a lightweight woollen fabric will do for any eventuality.

The Navy Blazer

The most versatile garment in your wardrobe. You can wear it with a shirt and tie just as easily as you can dress it down, wearing it with denim. The classic colour goes with pretty much everything – pale blue chambray, bright checks and prints – providing a contrast to softer shades.

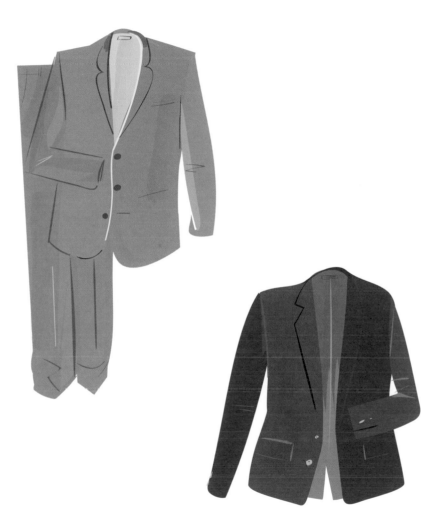

The Peacoat

The military outer-coat rooted in naval heritage – usually rendered in thick navy or black wool – with broad, double-breasted lapels, chunky buttons and vertical slash pockets. Worn slim, it's one of classic menswear's most versatile coats – a traditional men's piece that works with almost anything. Go traditional with a six-button closure and a cropped cut.

Denim Jeans

The traditional workwear garment that underwrites contemporary global style. Denim – the dark blue indigo-dyed tough cotton fabric – has countless permutations: special dyeing techniques, clever washes and hand treatments, or shot through with a little stretch. There is a growing industry in premium selvage denim (a traditionally made fabric with a tightly woven edge to prevent unravelling) often created in Japan on antique shuttle looms – and a preoccupation with historical workwear reimagined for modern times. Pick a dark indigo selvage denim in a slim, not skinny, cut. Consider a fabric with a tiny bit of stretch and hold off as long as you can between washes to help the indigo fade in a unique, characterful way. No bootcuts allowed.

The Denim Jacket

Another workwear classic, the durable denim jacket has been around since the late 1800s. Worn by the blue-collar workforce of America, denim jackets were frequently worn by cowboys and would go on to become firmly entrenched in popular culture.

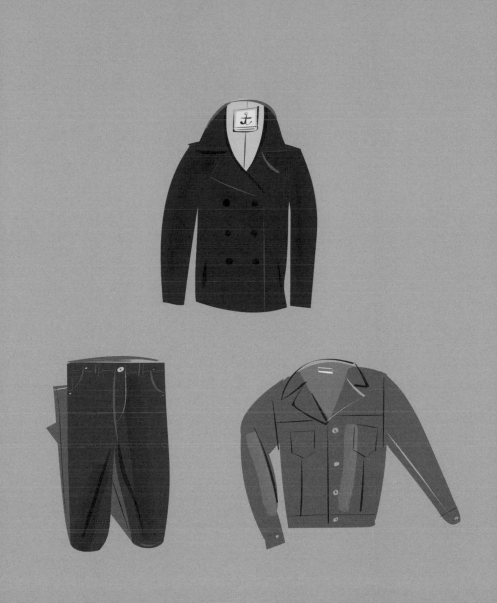

Punks, dweebs and bikers have all appropriated the denim jacket, and it now has classic garment status, with most major men's labels creating slim, trim versions. It dresses down any look, fits seamlessly into almost any outfit combination (even sweatpants) and – when worn with denim jeans – looks best if it's a different shade than what's down below.

The Chino

It might be a sign of getting older, but after a weekend watching a boxset in your sweat pants, a pair of ball-crushing skinny jeans just doesn't look comfortable any-more. Thank goodness, then, for the chino. Worn high-waisted by Diane Keaton in *Annie Hall*, baggy with a front pleat by Matthew Broderick in *Ferris Bueller's Day Off* and sported by David Hockney, 1980s heart-throb Nick Kamen and stylist Ray Petri's

Buffalo boys, the chino is as iconic as jeans, but with a level of comfort akin to wearing a skirt (I imagine). The most acquiescent of trouser styles looks good on almost anyone, even stretched over the buttocks of American tourists or Disney Store staffers. Few other garments have such cross-generational (and cross-gender) appeal – the chino's wrinkle-free, no-need-to-iron dependability would have your grandfather all aflutter.

The White Tee

Marlon Brando, before his shock weight gain and love affair with butter in *Last Tango in Paris*, was the iconic wearer of man's most important garment: the white T-shirt. And boy did he look cool. All bulges and brawn in *A Streetcar Named Desire* in 1951 (the classic film that cemented his stardom), and saucily grease-smudged in

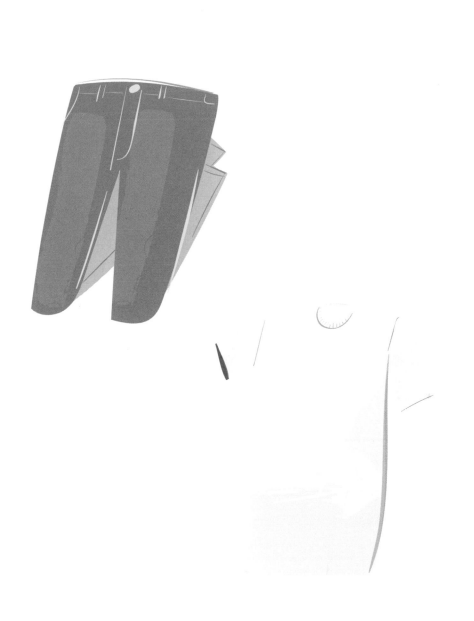

The Wild One in 1953, Brando unwittingly made the T-shirt the epitome of manliness. Still a staple of every man's wardrobe, for some reason it's near impossible to find a simple, unadulterated shirt of the like Brando might've cruised around the waterfront in. Menswear companies seem hellbent on splashing the humble tee with insipid graphics and almost-ironic slogans, none of which are quite as powerful or attractive as the plain, clean-living original. Worn underneath a collared shirt, it lends a cute, preppy look; under a Harrington jacket it's a tad modish and retro; and under a leather bomber, it's pure Brando – and, let's face it, a little Fonzie, too.

The Chambray Shirt

The (usually) pale blue, linen-finished, white weft cloth is a lightweight shirting staple. Worn with a knitted tie, or with a T-shirt underneath, this is the shirt that is truly versatile. Chambray is workwear, so look for quality and durability: off-white stitching, a soft surface and supple feel should be your checkpoints.

THE PREMIUM EXTRAS

Add these items to your wardrobe and they'll go with almost everything and anything: a plain crew-neck sweater in almost any colour – cotton knit or wool is best, and merino or cashmere is even better. Wear it with a simple white tee or even a button-down shirt underneath for a preppy look. A knitted tie fills in that tiny gap between smart-casual and formal, and brown leather shoes can be dressed up with a navy or grey suit or dressed down with dark denim jeans.

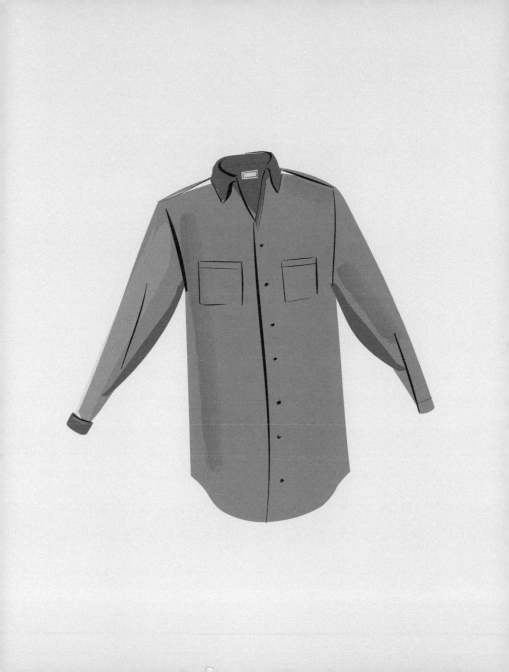

Icons of Grooming

MR FRANK OCEAN

A one-time ghostwriter for John Legend and
Justin Bieber (but don't let that put you off),
Mr Frank Ocean is the American singer-songwriter
and alt hip-hop impresario who is always
well-groomed. The hair-accessory supremo sports
a graphic tee or vintage shirt with a bandana
or headband tied tightly across his
forehead – a unique look, but somehow it works.

Style

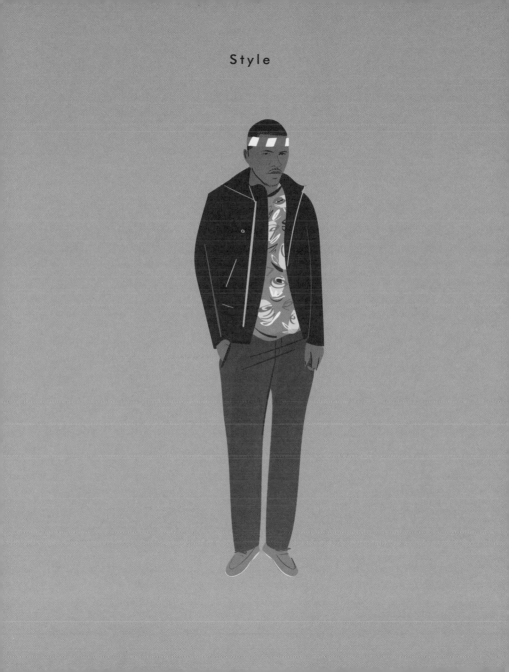

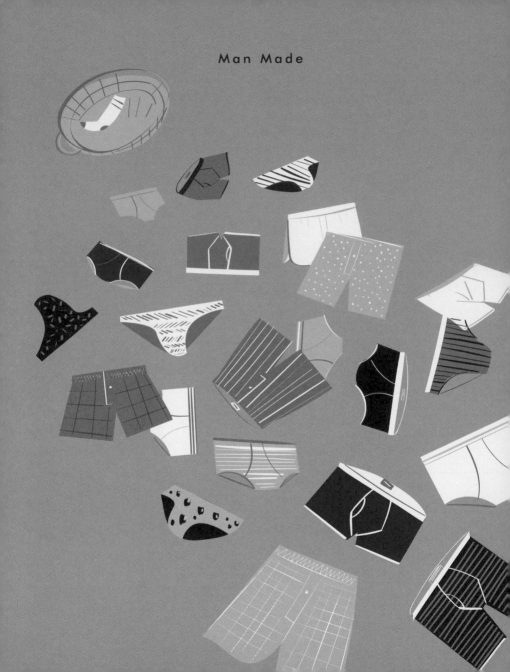

Man Made

How to Pick the Perfect Pair of Undies

The eternal conundrum: boxers or briefs? (Or boxer-briefs for those who like to sit, legs akimbo, on the fence.) When it's time to overhaul what you wear down there (undies seem to hold real nostalgia, and most of us have a few threadbare 'lucky' pairs on the go), there's a whole industry of underwear innovation to navigate. Some cling diligently to your private parts, holding and hoisting; Y-fronts and briefs, trunks and tangas all streamline and shape; while others let it all wobble free: voluminous boxers that offer no suggestion of what lurks within. A few tips to help you with your next nether-region style choice: pick natural over unnatural fabric (avoid 100 per cent nylon or polyester), erring towards cotton – even bamboo. Go for a classic navy or white or a subtle print, and pick a support style for sports and a slightly looser style for everyday shenanigans. Follow the sizing you use for jeans or chinos, pay attention to customer reviews and above all else: no Tweety Pie, Garfield or Simpsons cartoonery. Snoopy's okay.

CLASSIC BRANDS

There are a few iconic items that have achieved real cult status – and you could do worse than acquiring a few if not all of them.

RAY-BAN WAYFARERS

The American eyewear brand; hyper-cool since 1956. Tortoiseshell are ideal.

LEVI'S 501S

The US denim brand first introduced the 501 fit in 1890 – but it is the 1978 version that dominates.

CHUCK TAYLOR ALL-STARS

The cult off-white high-tops rendered in canvas and rubber, first produced in 1917, worn by anyone from the Ramones to Doctor Who.

HANES BEEFY-T

The budget tee with thick, flat ribbed collar and boxy fit. Stock up in white – and, if you can – pick up the Supreme collab version with its tiny, red printed Supreme tag.

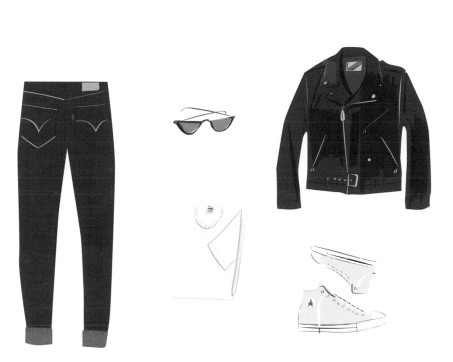

LEWIS LEATHERS BIKER JACKET

Dressing bikers since 1892, Lewis Leathers is Britain's oldest motorcycle clothing company. Pick up a second-hand vintage jacket for extra authenticity and sartorial credibility.

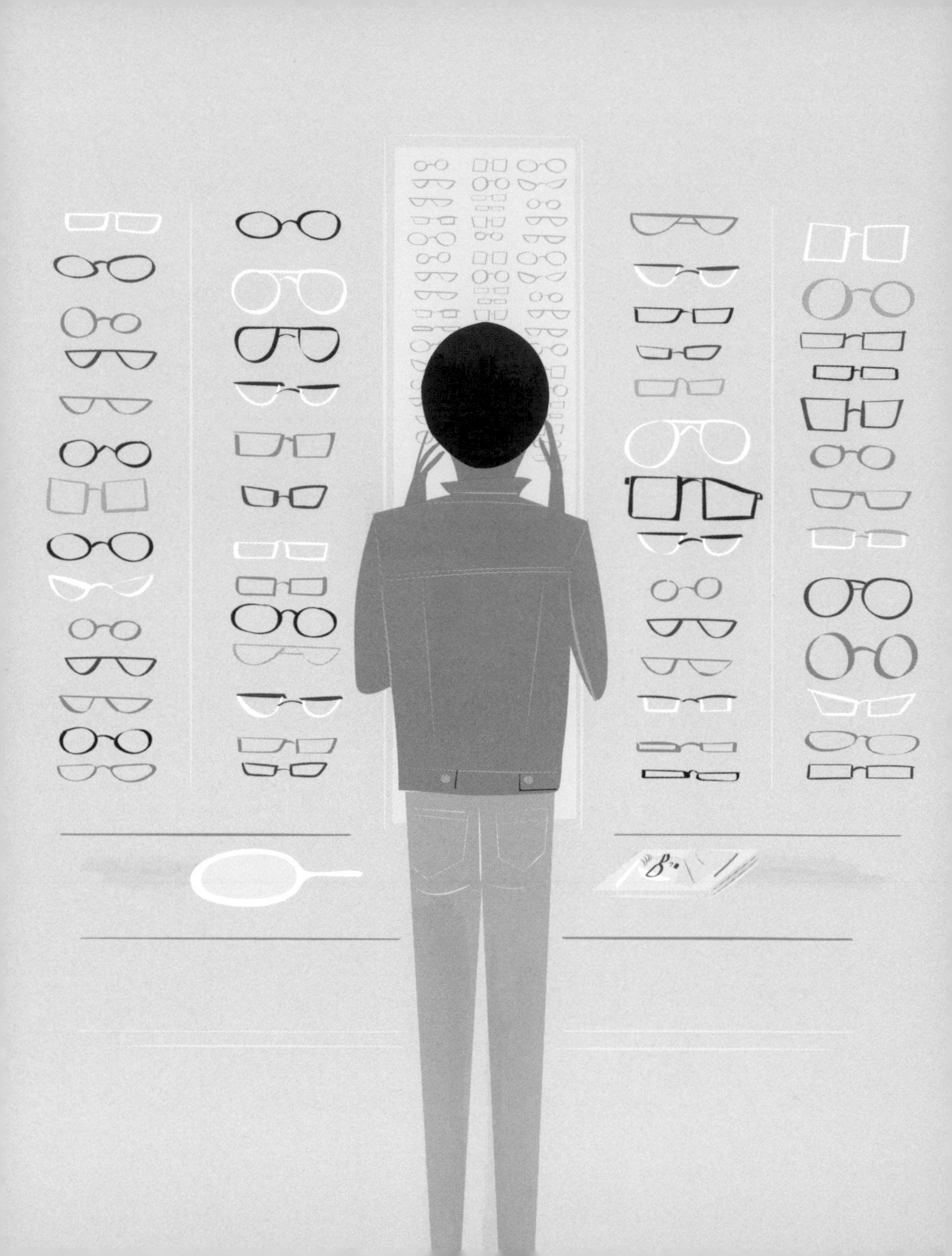

How to Buy Glasses

With an oval face shape generally considered to be the best proportion, glasses can help fool the eye into thinking that's just what you've got – even if you've got a mug like Frankenstein's monster. Round-faced people should generally avoid oval or circular styles (they'll make you look even rounder) and consider angular frames. Rectangular faces with high cheekbones and large foreheads are softened with wide frames (but avoid small square shapes). Or maybe you're a square with a wide forehead and jaw? Think about round or oval frames to take the edge off. Maybe you already have an oval face? If so, you can wear almost any style – lucky you. Ask an optician to help with frame size and lens shape, and think about what will clash or contrast with your hair or beard: bright red frames perched above a gingery handlebar moustache? It takes all sorts.

HOW TO SHOP

Men are supposed to hate shopping – I'm sure some do – but it's a shameless and rather sexist generalisation. Done right, shopping is creative, fun, speedy, and involves lunch out and an afternoon in the pub. Before shopping, clear out anything you don't wear; you can see where you've got gaps and plan what you're going to buy. Take a friend or two who'll warn you off buying anything too muttony, and get some honest feedback as you march out of the changing room. Work out what you're going to wear: if you're buying a suit wear a shirt, tie and your slickest leather shoes – if it's sneakers you're after, remember to wear socks (no one wants to wear those cheesy nanna's hold-ups they force you in 'for hygiene reasons'. Or is that just me?).

Speak up and question the assistant – visiting on a quieter day will mean you get their full attention. New-season stock usually arrives February and August, but be clever and anticipate the sales – in January and June, plus mid-season sales, pre-Christmas offers and Black Friday – now enjoyed almost everywhere across the globe. In a sense, it's easier to research a best price by shopping online – and any e-com retailer worth its salt should offer free delivery and returns, so you can always send back whatever you've invested in – no quibbles allowed.

HOW TO CARE FOR YOUR CLOTHES

Pick up your clothes from your hamper, peel them off the bedroom floor and empty out your gym bag into the nearest washing machine. As a rule, avoid super-hot washes – high heat will damage most fabrics – and try to pick a detergent that is free of dyes, fragrances and other nasties. It's almost as simple as that – apart from a few other important need-to-knows. Don't throw your

How to Fold a Shirt Perfectly Every Time

Button up the top and third buttons, lay the shirt face down (on a clean, hard surface), and smooth out any wrinkles. Starting on the left, fold about one third of the body of the shirt towards the centre (the fold should be from the centre of the left shoulder). Then, fold the left sleeve down with the cuff at the bottom; the sleeve should line up neatly to the edge of the first fold. Do the same the other side, and then fold up the shirttail a little – about a quarter of the way up the shirt. Finally, fold up again so the tail is just behind the collar. Flip over and… you're done.

Style

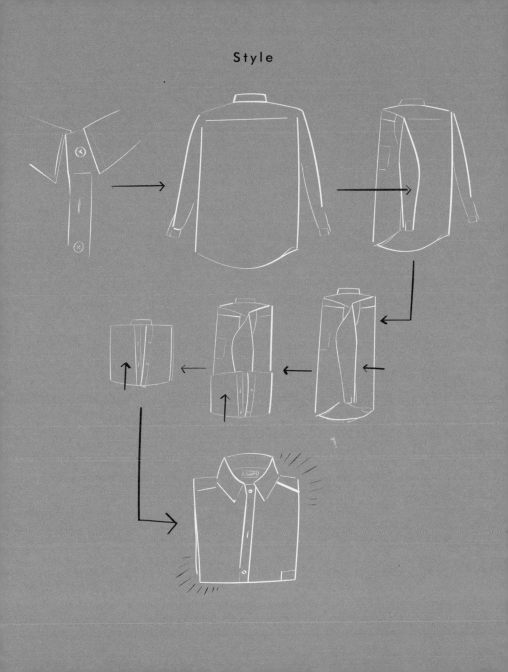

woollens into the washer. You need to dry-clean them, or hand wash with a special woollen detergent.

Dry-Cleaning

Dry-cleaning usually uses a cocktail of horrific chemicals (I usually don't bother – I'm not 100 per cent convinced my dry-cleaner does much more than just put my suit in a cupboard for a week) but there are eco-options. Ultimately, you should be caring for your clothing and dry-cleaning as little as possible. Never dry-clean a shirt, but wash or dry-clean a sweater every six wears or so, a cotton suit every two to three months (if you're wearing it most days) and a woollen suit about once a year.

Spritzing

Invest in a natural garment spray and freshen up all your clothes that don't spend all day nestling into your most intimate areas. It's a clever interim way to revive wool sweaters and suits, even denim – sort of like deodorant for your clothes.

Jean-cleaning

If you're the patient type, holding off that first wash on a new pair of dry denim jeans will create something completely unique. Premium, pared-down denim will transform into a super-faded fabric with high-contrast creases and cuts, scrapes and subtle abrasions – intense detail that will only reveal itself when jeans are finally washed and dried. But the longer you hold off that first wash, the more intense and individual the look. Original American denim brand Lee have a clever little wear counter – a simple way to tally up the days – printed inside the pocket lining of their premium Lee 101 jeans. You will be able to chart exactly how long you've worn your jeans before their first wash, and how long before their second dousing. When the time comes, fill your bath with a few inches of cold water and half a cup of wool wash (for dark woollens). Turn your jeans inside out and soak for ten minutes, then rinse with more cold water, and gently squeeze to remove most of the water. Finally, air- or sun-dry for about an hour and put them back on (still damp) if you want to retain their unique moulded-to-you shape.

Storing

Before hanging up your clothes, ramming them into drawers or squeezing them into bags – to be stored until the summer/winter – be sure everything you're storing is completely clean. Zip up your best suits in insect-proof, but not airtight, suit carriers, and give each garment – from a T-shirt to a ratty pair of undies – a little room to breathe.

Care Labels

Those odd symbols printed on the care instruction label of your favourite shirt, jacket or leather chaps? They actually do mean something. Here's a handy guide to decipher them:

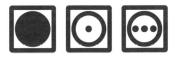

Wash temperature
One dot = cold;
three dots = hot

Dryer temperature
Black circle = no heat; one dot
= low; three dots = high

Bleach
Clear triangle
= it's safe

Dry-clean
Clear circle
= you can

Iron
One dot = low heat;
three dots = high

HOW TO POLISH YOUR SHOES

Much like the skin on your face, leather needs to be cleaned, nourished and protected. First up, remove dirt and dust with a bristle brush. Then, using an old rag, apply a few little dabs of leather conditioner in circular movements, really getting into those creases (this stage helps soften the leather in order to help it better absorb

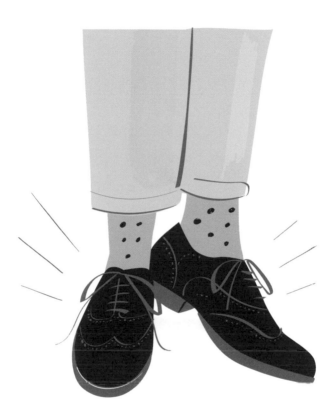

the polish). Allow the shoes to dry for a few minutes and then use a cream or wax polish in a colour that suits the shoe – ideally one slightly lighter than the leather so as not to darken the tone too noticeably. Apply with another old rag, in those steady circular motions, buff with a brush, and allow to dry.

Icons of Grooming

MR PATRICK GRANT

You'll not find a man more passionate about haberdashery than the perfectly turned-out Patrick Grant. He is the British designer and creative director of tailors Norton & Sons, credited with transforming the fortunes of another men's brand, E. Tautz. The word 'suave' – dripping with cliché – should only be used very rarely.
Describing Mr Patrick Grant is one such time.

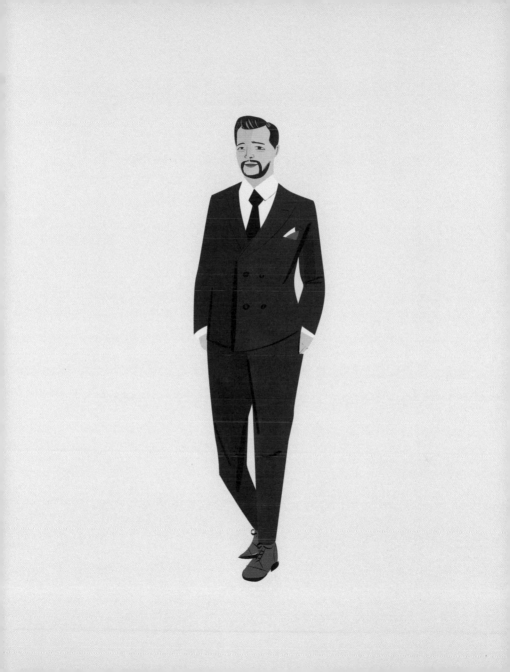

THE BATHROOM CABINET

There are all manner of odd things in my bathroom cabinet: a flea-market toothbrush mug that commemorates Charles & Di's wedding, almost-empty cologne bottles from yesteryear, Disney Princess Elastoplast, and a tube of something for that weird rash I had that time. But there are also the 15 most important grooming products I've ever used. I have tried and tested each one – sometimes for years – and they're all 100 per cent excellent. I'd look and smell at least 96 years old without them.

15 FAILSAFE GROOMING PRODUCTS

LUCAS' PAWPAW OINTMENT

Gungy and gloopy, Lucas' Pawpaw Ointment is the cult all-purpose Australian product unchanged for more 100 years. Using fruit grown and fermented in sunny Queensland, it's excellent as a lip balm, but also for dry skin and sunburn, and –

being naturally bacterial – you can use it on burns, chaffing and even small cuts and grazes.

AESOP GERANIUM LEAF BODY BALM

Founded in Melbourne in 1987, Aesop products – packaged in simple medicinal brown bottles – achieve a clever balance between plant-based elements and lab-made ingredients of super-powered quality. Who cares when the products smell and feel as good as the Aesop Geranium Leaf Body Balm? Sniffing this is like a legal high and the super rich cream really hydrates the skin.

BURT'S BEES SUPER SHINY MANGO SHAMPOO

Natural, sustainable, and just a little hippy-edged Burt's Bees is the skin, hair and bodycare brand that's wild about ecology and bees.

Its Super Shiny mango shampoo, packed with mango seed oil and fig extract, is the fruit salad of hair cleansers, moisturising and reducing frizz like no other. It gives me a real buzz (see what I did there?) to say that the accompanying conditioner is great, too.

KIEHL'S CALENDULA DEEP CLEANSING FOAMING FACE WASH

Kiehl's, once an old-world pharmacy, was founded in 1851 in Manhattan's East Village, peddling clever treatments, homemade remedies, and the first own brand name products. Today, its super-science-meets-natural ingredients approach – powered by the brand's owners, L'Oreal – means Kiehl's products have a powerful effect. The Kiehl's Calendula Foaming Face Wash is a brilliant, soap-free gel with a simple fragrance that is great for normal to oily skin.

DERMALOGICA SKIN PREP SCRUB

One of my favourite brands, Dermalogica is the indie skincare outfit that formulates without irritants (mineral oil, lanolin, artificial colours and fragrances) and focuses on 'skin health fitness' and high-performance formulas over packaging and hype. Its Skin Prep Scrub is a mild exfoliant powered by corncob meal and is gentle enough to use two to three times a week. I reach for this when I know I'm looking a bit lacklustre and it always perks my skin up.

DR BRONNER'S MAGIC 'ALL-ONE' SOAP

Organic, fair trade, mostly vegan, and all completely natural, indie brand Dr Bronner's magical soaps have many uses, but washing your skin is probably the most common. Top flavours include Patchouli, Almond, and Peppermint (which certainly leaves a magical tingle in certain places). Read the late Doc's leftfield philosophy – handily printed on product labels – to discover his mystical approach to keeping clean.

DERMALOGICA ACTIVE MOIST

Active Moist is the moisturiser I use every single day, without fail. Lightweight and oil-free, it's more of a lotion than a cream – and a little goes a long, long way. Packed with silk amino acids, your post-wash skin drinks it up in seconds, leaving a fresh, clean feel. To maintain the super-light consistency, there's no built-in sun protection so remember to apply your own.

KIEHL'S MIDNIGHT RECOVERY EYE

An effective eye cream that melts into the skin working on puffiness, fine lines, and wrinkles. The clue's in the name: as it's rich, Kiehl's Midnight Recovery Eye is supposed to be used overnight, but you can use it during the day. It's fragrance-free with no Parabens or mineral oils – just a little Butchers Broom, Evening Primrose oil and Lavender – making it powerful and pretty much irritant free.

MURDOCK LONDON BEARD MOISTURISER

This award-winning Beard Moisturiser is truly brilliant. The London-based men's grooming brand – and chain of excellent barbershops – has a full range of luxury gent's essentials, all of which smell otherworldly. Its Beard Moisturiser is no exception: packed with Aloe Vera, Eucalyptus

and Menthol, it' a powerful conditioner for bristly beards.

TOM FORD PRIVATE BLEND TUSCAN LEATHER EAU DE PARFUM

This is the most properly luxurious fragrance I've ever owned. Tom Ford Private Blend Tuscan Leather Eau de Parfum is a blend of rare, high-grade perfume oils that smell like a premium leather shoe emporium. Only better. It's a rich, evocative aroma with raspberry, saffron, thyme and jasmine notes and, being an Eau de Parfum, it's also rather expensive – but extremely potent and lasts for ages.

COMME DES GARÇONS X MONOCLE LAUREL

Leftfield fashion brand Comme des Garçons worked with upscale media outfit Monocle to create a fragrance inspired by the Lebanon. They set out to try and recreate the 'distinctive scent of laurel that punctuated an early spring weekend in the eastern Mediterranean' and they nailed it. This super fresh, zingy aroma smells just like crushed up laurel leaves – it's like catnip for humans.

ESTÉE LAUDER IDEALIST PORE MINIMIZING SKIN REFINISHER

The big secret. This powerful little product is marketed to women, but it doesn't discriminate in its skin super-powers. The Idealist Pore Minimizing Skin Refinisher is an unbelievably potent serum that shrinks your pores leaving you clear, clean and smooth looking, and makes your face feel impossibly silky and smooth in just one go. Highly recommended.

KIEHL'S STYLIST SERIES CRÈME WITH SILK GROOM

Yet another Kiehl's star product, if you're using a hair cream for a bit of light hold and shine, this should be your go-to (especially if you have wavy hair). It moisturises and conditions, and added silk powders and oils add real softness and shine to your hair without a greasy feel. Apply to damp hair and rake through with your fingers, adding a tiny bit more when dry to define. A real frizz-tamer.

EDWIN JAGGER CHROME LINED DOUBLE-EDGE SAFETY RAZOR

Most of us use disposable razors and for good reason: brands like Gilette make excellent multi-blade products that do the job perfectly, but they usually err away from

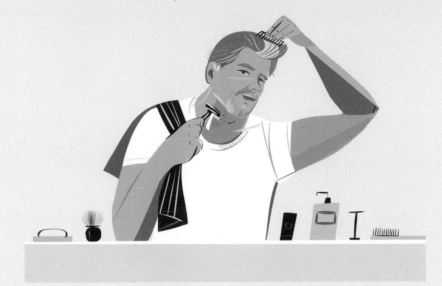

simple, strong (and traditional) design. Like Merkur, Edwin Jagger is a great British brand that creates sturdy, great looking and pleasingly weighty razors that fill the gap.

BLACK & WHITE ORIGINAL PLUKO HAIR POMADE

The low cost cult classic that's been knocking around a chemist or drugstore near you for more than 90 years. Black & White Original Pluko Hair Pomade is fantastic at giving a high-shine effect with a light hold, and smells nothing short of amazing. Unlike most pomades, it washes out easily and it's best for slightly wavy hair (it's not strong enough to tame very curly hair). Also, it's shockingly cheap.

Biographies

DAN JONES

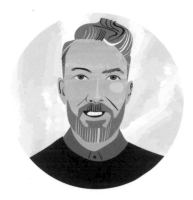

Style and grooming writer Dan Jones was born in 1977, the year *Never Mind The Bollocks, Here's The Sex Pistols* was released. He has lived and worked in London and Sydney and tried and tested almost every haircut known to man, from Morrissey pompadours to mermaid hair streaks. His favourite movie moustache is worn by Serpico era Al Pacino, and most beloved beard is a hair's breadth between Hagrid and Steve Zissou.

LIBBY VANDERPLOEG

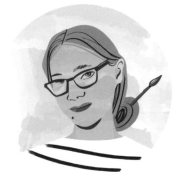

Born in Michigan on the edge of the great lakes, Libby VanderPloeg is an illustrator currently living and working in Greenpoint, Brooklyn. She enjoys drawing and painting flora and fauna of all varieties, and prefers to work with a strong cup of coffee always at arm's reach. Her work has been featured in such publications as The Wall Street Journal, The Boston Globe, and Design*Sponge, and in books published by Farrar, Straus & Giroux and HarperCollins.

Acknowledgements

Big hairy thanks to publisher Kate Pollard, pocket rocket editor Kajal Mistry, and all at Hardie Grant, plus tough sub editor Zelda Turner. The most excellent art direction of Matt Phare really made this book look its best – like it's just stepped out of a salon. And then there's illustrator, artist, and spiritual bearded lady Libby Vanderploeg: my transatlantic co-pilot, who turned words into pictures in ways I hadn't even imagined. This book is the culmination of years of awful hairstyles, style slip-ups, and indescribable skin complaints until I got into my groove with the input of some world-class skin, health, and fashion experts.

And I'll forever be grateful to have the hirsute advice of my favourite barbers in the world: Tom Bushnell of Folk Barber, Steve Murphy and Neil Scothon of Rocket Barbers, Mr Ducktail of It's Something Hell's, and all at Murdock London.

Man Made

Index

Index

Man Made by Dan Jones

First published in 2015 by Hardie Grant Books

Hardie Grant Books (UK)
5th & 6th Floors
52–54 Southwark Street
London SE1 1UN
www.hardiegrant.co.uk

Hardie Grant Books (Australia)
Ground Floor, Building 1
658 Church Street
Melbourne, VIC 3121
www.hardiegrant.com.au

British Library Cataloguing-in-Publication Data. A catalogue record
for this book is available from the British Library.

ISBN: 978-1-78488-013-2

Publisher: Kate Pollard
Senior Editor: Kajal Mistry
Art Direction: Matt Phare
Illustrator © Libby VanderPloeg
Editor: Zelda Turner
Proofreaders: Lorraine Jerram and Louise Francis
Indexer: Cathy Heath
Colour Reproduction by p2d

Printed and bound in China by 1010

10 9 8 7 6 5 4 3 2 1

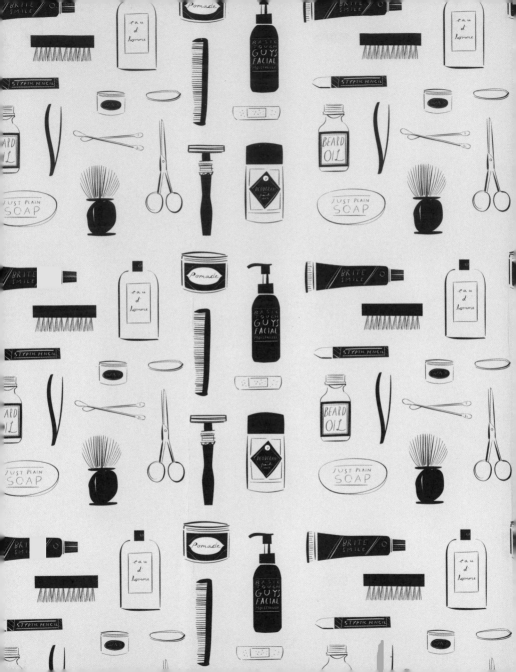